Schizophrenia
Innovations in Diagnosis and Treatment

Colin A. Ross, MD

HMTP

The Haworth Maltreatment and Trauma Press®
An Imprint of The Haworth Press, Inc.
New York • London • Oxford

Published by

The Haworth Maltreatment and Trauma Press®, an imprint of The Haworth Press, Inc., 10 Alice Street, Binghamton, NY 13904-1580.

Chapter 6 by John Read and Colin A. Ross (2003) was previously published as "Psychological Trauma and Psychosis" in the *Journal of the American Academy of Psychoanalysis and Dynamic Psychiatry,* 31(1): 247-268. Reprinted by permission of The Guilford Press.

Excerpts from *Dementia Praecox or the Group of Schizophrenias* by Eugen Bleuler are reprinted by permission of International Universities Press, Inc. Copyright 1950 by International Universities Press.

Excerpt from Sheila Cantor (1988), *Childhood Schizophrenia,* p. 1, reprinted by permission of The Guilford Press.

PUBLISHER'S NOTE
Identities and circumstances of individuals discussed in this book have been changed to protect confidentiality.

Cover design by Marylouise E. Doyle.

Library of Congress Cataloging-in-Publication Data

Ross, Colin A.
  Schizophrenia : innovations in diagnosis and treatment / Colin A. Ross.
    p. ; cm.
Includes bibliographical references and index.
  ISBN 0-7890-2269-9 (hard : alk. paper)—ISBN 0-7890-2270-2 (soft : alk. paper)
  1. Schizophrenia—Diagnosis. 2. Schizophrenia—Treatment. 3. Dissociative disorders.
  [DNLM: 1. Dissociative Disorders. 2. Schizophrenia. WM 203 R823s 2004] I. Title.

RC514.R67 2004
616.89'8075—dc22

2004000374

Colin A. Ross, MD

Schizophrenia
Innovations in Diagnosis and Treatment

"*Schizophrenia: Innovations in Diagnosis and Treatment* is an original, important, and thought-provoking contribution to the study of schizophrenia and dissociation and their relation to trauma. In 2004, psychiatry is increasingly oriented to biology and psychopharmacology. Psychiatry's fascination with the brain threatens to obscure its appreciation of the mind, and its obsession with the gene tempts it to overlook the contributions of life experiences to mental illness. Colin Ross offers a timely and trenchant analysis of the limitations of the paradigm of biological psychiatry. Colin Ross is reductionistic biological psychiatry's Michael Moore, using its own words and data to demonstrate its myopia, shortcomings, and self-deceptions. He moves beyond this critique to engage the reader in a more rich and nuanced study of psychosis and dissociation, the relationship between them, and the role of trauma in the development of psychopathology. Whether or not the reader agrees with Ross's concept of a dissociative subtype of schizophrenia and his proposals for its treatment, the reader cannot avoid being moved by his plea that an effort should be made to understand patients more completely and to provide them with care that responds not to the dominant theories of the day, but to the clinical realities of their conditions."

Richard P. Kluft, MD
Clinical Professor of Psychiatry,
Temple University School of Medicine;
Past President, ISSD

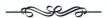

"This is a scholarly, well-documented, and clearly explained treatise with hugely significant implications for our diagnostic system and for how severely disturbed people are understood and treated. Dr. Ross transcends the simplistic biogenetic ideology that so often clouds our thinking about madness to bring us a truly evidence-based approach to understanding schizophrenia. Fifteen years ago Dr. Ross was among the first to break psychiatry's shameful silence about child abuse and psychosis. He now develops his groundbreaking theory to explain just how, and how often, childhood trauma can lead to madness.

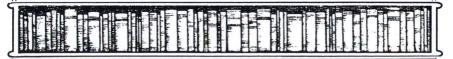

More pre-publication
REVIEWS, COMMENTARIES, EVALUATIONS . . .

Dr. Ross's prediction that 25 to 40 percent of individuals currently diagnosed with schizophrenia have the dissociative, trauma-based subtype of the disorder will cause consternation among biologically oriented psychiatrists. It may well, however, turn out to be an underestimate."

John Read, PhD
Editor, *Models of Madness: Psychological, Social and Biological Approaches to Schizophrenia*
Director of Clinical Psychology, The University of Auckland

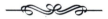

"In *Schizophrenia: An Innovative Approach to Diagnosis and Treatment*, Colin Ross, MD, an international authority on dissociative disorders, exposes a major failure of modern psychiatry. Although a century ago, Bleuler, the grand old master of schizophrenia, observed extensive dissociation and trauma in many of his patients, mainstream psychiatry is either ignorant of or unwilling to acknowledge current clinical observations and empirical research that confirm those pioneering observations. Based on recent findings and using careful reasoning, Ross convincingly argues that a significant proportion of schizophrenic patients suffer from what he coins as a subtype of dissociative schizophrenia—a proposed diagnosic category that straddles schizophrenia and the dissociative disorders. As a rule, these patients report extensive trauma histories and are refractory to traditional treatment, i.e., medication. Trauma-related symptoms in dissociative schizophrenic patients are often phenomenologically analogous to psychotic symptoms but are responsive to appropriate psychotherapy. Such treatment can lead to significant functional improvement in this subgroup rather than simply attempting to teach them to manage a chronic mental illness. Readers open to the message of this book cannot help but conclude that current psychiatric practice is doing these patients much harm by treating them insufficiently and inappropriately. At the very least, the application of Ross's innovative approach, which is firmly rooted in phase-oriented treatment of complex trauma-related disorders, should greatly reduce iatrogenic damage.

This book is a *must* for all clinicians and researchers dealing with serious mental disorders. Students in the various mental health disciplines are strongly recommended to read this book, thereby preventing themselves from copying traditional views that have been so detrimental to patients suffering from dissociative schizophrenia."

Onno van der Hart, PhD
Professor of Psychopathology of Chronic Traumatization,
Department of Clinical Psychology,
Utrecht University, Utrecht,
the Netherlands

HMTP

The Haworth Maltreatment and Trauma Press®
An Imprint of The Haworth Press, Inc.
New York • London • Oxford

Schizophrenia
Innovations in Diagnosis and Treatment

As in almost *all* disease forms with which we deal, including the plainly exogenous ones, we are far from dealing with simple etiological constellations in the mental disorders of the deterioration group. The main contrasts or extremes are the cases with strong constitutional bias requiring but little extraneous cause— and those with at least superficially more normal makeup and a preponderance of overt more or less extraneous or circumstantial etiological factors.

Adolph Meyer
The Nature and Conception of Dementia Praecox, 1911

It is likely that schizophrenia is the final common pathway for a group of disorders with a variety of etiologies, courses, and outcomes. To provide more-precise diagnosis and prognosis and more-specific treatment approaches, it would be helpful if subgroups of patients with schizophrenia were identified.

American Psychiatric Association
Practice Guideline for the Treatment
of Patients with Schizophrenia, 1997

ABOUT THE AUTHOR

Colin A. Ross, MD, has been supervising an inpatient program for psychological trauma in Dallas since 1991. Dr. Ross is a former Associate Professor in the Department of Psychiatry at the University of Manitoba. He is a past President of the International Society for the Study of Dissociation and has received several awards from the organization. He currently consults to and supervises trauma programs at hospitals in Texas, California, and Michigan. He is also a member of the International Society for the Psychological Treatment of Schizophrenia and Other Psychoses (ISPS) and has served on an ISPS Task Force on psychosocial treatments of schizophrenia.

Dr. Ross is Founder and President of the Colin A. Ross Institute for Psychological Trauma (www.rossinst.com), which provides treatment, consultation, training, and education concerning psychological trauma and its consequences. He has published numerous journal papers, books, book chapters, and essays dealing with psychological trauma, dissociation, and psychosis. He is also the owner of Manitou Communications, a multimedia publishing company that produces books, videos, and CDs on trauma-related topics.

CONTENTS

Preface

I remember watching the film *Lilith* many years ago and being very impressed by the scene in which a psychiatrist shows pictures of alarming, disorganized webs woven by psychotic spiders. I learned while doing research for this book that the scene was based on the work of Bercel (1959), who injected serum from schizophrenic patients into spiders. It seems certain to me that many people with schizophrenia must have a biological disease of some kind. Their brains just don't seem to work properly.

On the other hand, I have worked with many individuals who have a different diagnosis: dissociative identity disorder (DID), formerly called multiple personality disorder (Ross, 1989, 1994, 1995, 1997, 2000a,b). These people hear voices, have delusional thinking, and experience many of the classical Schneiderian symptoms of schizophrenia, but they are different. Though two-thirds meet structured interview criteria for schizoaffective disorder or schizophrenia, they can often achieve integration, at which time their psychoses go into long-term remission.

Although they are psychotic by the criteria of the *Diagnostic and Statistical Manual of Mental Disorders,* Fourth Edition, Text Revision (DSM-IV-TR) (American Psychiatric Association, 2000) and score high on all measures of psychosis, people with DID are different from those with schizophrenia. Their symptoms seem to be predominantly a reaction to the environment, and they are treatable with psychotherapy. It is obvious to me, from my clinical experience, that many people with schizophrenia cannot be treated with psychotherapy.

What is the problem, then? We have two distinct diagnoses, listed in distinct sections of the DSM-IV-TR: schizophrenia and DID. DID is a reaction to the environment that is treatable with psychotherapy; schizophrenia is a biological brain disease treated with medications. End of discussion, one would think.

For current diagnosis, treatment, and research on schizophrenia, it is the end of the discussion. The schizophrenia field is untouched by the literature on trauma and dissociation. For instance, childhood sexual abuse and dissociation are not mentioned once in a book that gives considerable attention to the problem of nature versus nurture in schizophrenia (Gottesman, 1991) or in a recent review article on schizophrenia (Goff, 2002).

The reverse is not true, however. The relationship between dissociation and psychosis, multiple personality disorder and schizophrenia has been a subject of serious thought as well as clinical and research attention in the dissociative disorders field for over twenty years (Bliss, 1980; Fink and Golinkoff, 1990; Gainer, 1994; Kluft, 1987; Laddis et al., 2001; Putnam, 1989; Rosenbaum, 1980; Ross, 1997; Steinberg et al., 1994; Van der Hart, Witztum, and Friedman, 1993). In the dissociative disorders field, the differential diagnosis of DID and schizophrenia is a complex and important problem, with major implications for treatment and prognosis.

If an individual receives a diagnosis of schizophrenia in the United States today, treatment will consist primarily of medication with adjunctive social support and education about the biological nature of the illness. There will be no intensive, long-term individual psychotherapy. However, if the same person receives a diagnosis of DID, the primary treatment will be psychotherapy; medications will be adjunctive. Antidepressants and anxiolytics will be prescribed more often than neuroleptics.

In the schizophrenia field, this is not a problem because DID is not considered in the differential diagnosis, and intensive psychotherapy is not considered in the treatment plan. However, the problem exists in the dissociative disorders field. I have worked with many individuals who previously received diagnoses of schizoaffective disorder or schizophrenia for whom I made a diagnosis of DID. These people participate in individual long-term psychotherapy as effectively as any I have ever met.

It is now twenty-five years since I diagnosed my first case of multiple personality disorder as a medical student and twenty years since I published the case (Ross, 1984). The woman, my first psychotherapy patient, has been integrated for more than a decade. During this period of twenty-five years, I have seen only a small shift in the attitude of psychiatrists toward DID and the other dissociative disorders. It seems unlikely that the field of psychiatry is going to allocate significant academic, teaching, research, or clinical resources to DID in the near future.

This is a problem, from my perspective, because many people in treatment for schizophrenia could benefit from psychotherapy for DID. There is very little chance that their diagnoses will be revised to DID if they are being treated for schizophrenia and very little chance they will be offered intensive psychotherapy if they continue to receive the diagnosis of schizophrenia.

My solution to this problem is to propose the existence of a dissociative subtype of schizophrenia. This is not simply a political or tactical move; I propose that dissociative schizophrenia is a valid and reliable subtype of the disorder. Its existence is supported by clinical and research literature extending back to Bleuler (1950 [1911]) and its diagnostic criteria can be operationalized and tested scientifically.

Using DSM-IV-TR criteria, the same individual can receive diagnoses of both DID and schizophrenia because DSM-IV-TR rules do not make either an exclusion criterion for the other. Clinicians may diagnose DID if they prefer, or schizophrenia, or both. Because far more psychiatrists are willing to make a diagnosis of schizophrenia than of DID, individuals who meet criteria for both DID and schizophrenia (or schizoaffective disorder) are much more likely to receive a diagnosis of psychosis.

The problem could be solved if DID was included within the category of dissociative schizophrenia, but it would be premature to suggest this change to the DSM-IV-TR system in 2004. The proposal would not be accepted by either the dissociative disorders field or the schizophrenia field at present; it lacks conclusive empirical evidence, and it has not been subjected to professional discussion and criticism.

The purpose of the dissociative subtype of schizophrenia, at a practical level, is to allow clinicians to recognize the role of trauma and dissociation in a subgroup of individuals who meet DSM-IV-TR criteria for both schizophrenia and a dissociative disorder, without having to make a diagnosis of DID or dissociative disorder not otherwise specified (DDNOS). Also, it opens up the possibility of an environmental etiology for a major subtype of schizophrenia and would stimulate research on classification, etiology, phenomenology, psychobiology, psychopharmacology, and psychotherapy of the subtype. Psychiatry has closed the door on the psychotherapy of schizophrenia. We need to reopen that door, go through it, and conduct serious, sustained studies in that neglected territory.

I propose that we have in the dissociative disorders field a minutely detailed, operationalized, and effective treatment for a subtype of schizophrenia—a hypothesis worthy of serious study. I agree with the Patient Outcomes Research Team (PORT) (Lehman and Steinwachs, 1998) recommendation that psychotherapies focused on transference and regression are contraindicated in schizophrenia, and I agree that the psychotherapy of schizophrenia should focus on cognitive, behavioral, educational, and supportive strategies and principles. However, I believe that psychodynamic principles are also useful and should not be excluded.

In *Schizophrenia: Innovations in Diagnosis and Treatment* I attempt to define a subgroup of individuals within the DSM-IV-TR category of schizophrenia who are more likely to respond to psychotherapy, who are more likely to report severe childhood trauma, and who have more extensive comorbidity. The hypothesis of a dissociative subtype of schizophrenia serves several functions: to call attention to the need for serious study of dissociation in the schizophrenia field; to provide a structure for future investigations; to call for a reconsideration of the role of psychotherapy in schizophrenia; and to propose that there is a valid dissociative subtype of the disorder. The heuristic goals of the hypothesis can be met even if the validity of the subtype is not accepted or incorporated in future editions of the DSM.

I suggest that 25 to 40 percent of individuals currently in treatment for schizophrenia have the dissociative subtype of the disorder. I have seen people in treatment for DID who meet structured interview and DSM-IV-TR criteria for schizoaffective disorder or schizophrenia respond very well to psychotherapy, with stable, long-term remission of their auditory hallucinations. There is real hope for recovery for people with the dissociative subtype of schizophrenia. The purpose of this book is to present all the reasons for taking that proposition seriously.

Acknowledgments

Schizophrenia: Innovations in Diagnosis and Treatment questions the endogenous biomedical disease model of schizophrenia, the efficacy of antipsychotic medication, the clear separation of schizophrenia from dissociative disorders, and the belief that schizophrenia has nothing to do with childhood trauma. I am indebted to those who have offered encouragement and support for my study of trauma, dissociation, and psychosis, given its controversial nature. The criticisms and suggestions of the anonymous reviewer of the manuscript were extremely helpful. The book is better organized and argued because of the reviewer's input.

I included a section on Schneiderian first-rank symptoms of schizophrenia in the Dissociative Disorders Interview Schedule (Ross, 1997) that I created in 1986, and I included Schneiderian symptoms in a questionnaire about multiple personality disorder that I mailed out in 1987 (Ross, Norton, and Wozney, 1989). It has been clear to me since medical school that the relationship between multiple personality disorder and schizophrenia is a complex problem, and that its solution challenges the endogenous biomedical disease model of schizophrenia.

I am indebted to four colleagues who wrote articles on this problem (Bliss, 1980; Gainer, 1994; Kluft, 1987; Rosenbaum, 1980). These four articles helped me with my thinking and with my resolve to study this problem carefully.

More recently, members of the International Society for the Psychological Treatments of the Schizophrenias and Other Psychoses (ISPS) have provided encouragement, support, and rational criticism (Ross, in press). Foremost among these colleagues is John Read—his articles mark the first time I saw my research and thinking about trauma and psychosis taken seriously in the psychiatric literature. I would like to thank my fellow members of the ISPS task force set up to respond to the recommendations concerning psychotherapy for schizophrenia in the Schizophrenia Patient Outcomes Research Team

Report (Lehman and Steinwachs, 1998). I learned a lot from participation in the task force.

Articles resulting from the ISPS task force (Bachmann, Resch, and Mundt, 2003; Gleeson, Larsen, and McGorry, 2003; Gottdiener and Haslam, 2003; Larsen, Bechdolf, and Birchwood, 2003; Margison, 2003; Read and Ross, 2003) appear in a special issue of the *Journal of the American Academy of Psychoanalysis and Dynamic Therapy,* edited by Silver and Larsen (2003). These are supplemented by a number of additional articles on the psychotherapy of schizophrenia, including further commentary by Lehman and Steinwachs (2003).

Chapter 6 of this book is a modified version of an article by John Read and myself (Read and Ross, 2003). Several paragraphs from that work are included in Chapter 4 as well. This material is reproduced with permission of The Guilford Press. Chapter 7 is a revised version of the appendix to my book *The Trauma Model* (Ross, 2000b). This material is reproduced with the permission of Manitou Communications.

Since its inception in 1984, I have received support from the International Society for the Study of Dissociation (ISSD). The society has provided a forum for me to present my ideas and research data at meetings and in print. No other professional organization has provided even a fraction of the support I have received from the ISSD.

Finally, I would like, as always, to thank my teachers—my patients. They have taught me that auditory hallucinations, Schneiderian passivity experiences, delusions, and other symptoms of psychosis can be environmentally induced and can be treatable with psychotherapy. This is true, I have learned, even among individuals who meet DSM-IV-TR and structured interview criteria for schizophrenia or schizoaffective disorder.

A Statement of the Problem

Schizophrenia: Innovations in Diagnosis and Treatment defines a set of problems in psychiatry. My goal is to get these problems recognized within the mental health field and the culture as a whole. By recognized I mean seen, understood, taken seriously, and invested in. By invested in I mean that these problems should receive time, money, energy, and priority in the mental health field.

The interrelated set of problems is as follows:

1. The pendulum of psychiatry in the United States has swung too far toward endogenous biomedical models of schizophrenia.
2. Too much emphasis is placed on medication in the treatment of schizophrenia and too little on psychotherapy.
3. Too much emphasis is placed on genetic causes of schizophrenia and too little on environmental causes.
4. The scientific data do not support a primarily genetic cause of schizophrenia.
5. The scientific data support the conclusion that antipsychotic medications are only modestly effective.
6. The epidemiology and phenomenology of chronic, complex dissociative disorders are poorly understood by most psychiatrists.
7. A great deal of overlap exists between dissociation and psychosis—this is true at the levels of phenomenology, DSM-IV-TR diagnostic criteria, and measurement of symptoms.
8. The overlap between dissociation and psychosis is not recognized in the schizophrenia field.
9. The overlap between dissociation and psychosis is much more than a problem of unrecognized comorbidity; many of the core features of schizophrenia and DID are the same. For instance, positive symptoms of schizophrenia are more characteristic of DID than they are of schizophrenia. DSM-IV-TR

diagnostic criteria, structured diagnostic interviews, and symptom measures cannot differentiate the two disorders in many cases, and clinicians frequently cannot differentiate the two disorders. As well, unrecognized cases of DID are readily apparent in Eugen Bleuler's (1950 [1911]) text, *Dementia Praecox or the Group of Schizophrenias*.

10. The overlap between the core features of DID and schizophrenia cannot be reduced to a problem of comorbidity because the two disorders are not discrete and separate categories. They cannot be comorbid with each other because they are too often and too much the same thing.

The first step in solving these problems is to get them recognized and taken seriously. That is my primary goal in this book. The second step is to propose possible solutions:

1. Define a model of the brain-mind field that allows for causality of serious mental disorders to run in two directions: brain to mind and mind to brain.
2. Define an operationalized dissociative subtype of schizophrenia.
3. Provide measures and methodology for demonstrating the reliability and validity of the dissociative subtype of schizophrenia.
4. Propose two alternative schemes for the relationship between the dissociative subtype of schizophrenia and chronic, complex dissociative disorders, principally DID.
5. Review the relevant literature and data supporting the existence of a dissociative subtype of schizophrenia.

The ultimate goals of this book are as follows:

1. Stimulate serious research on the psychotherapy of schizophrenia.
2. Stimulate serious research on the environmental causes of schizophrenia, principally severe childhood psychological trauma.
3. Stimulate recognition of the major role of dissociation in the phenomenology of a substantial subset of individuals with schizophrenia.

If these goals are met, I will be more than satisfied.

PART I:
A DISSOCIATIVE SUBTYPE
OF SCHIZOPHRENIA

Chapter 1

Assumptions and Logic Underlying the Dissociative Subtype of Schizophrenia

Within psychiatry, there is virtually unanimous adherence to the biopsychosocial model of mental illness. The theory of a dissociative subtype of schizophrenia is rooted in a biopsychosocial approach that gives equal etiological weight, in principle, to the biological, the psychological, and the social. Biological variables in dissociative schizophrenia are no more important, fundamental, scientific, or medical than psychological ones. *Genotype* in this chapter means a segment or segments of abnormal DNA with a causal and diagnostically specific relationship to the schizophrenia phenotype.

This chapter outlines the assumptions and logic that underlie the theory of a dissociative subtype of schizophrenia. The empirical foundations of the subtype are presented in later chapters. Throughout this book, I use the terms *dissociative subtype of schizophrenia* and *dissociative schizophrenia* interchangeably.

The phenomenology, reliability, and validity of dissociative schizophrenia can be established only by empirical investigation, but, as is done in all areas of science, I have pursued this line of investigation and study on the basis of intuition, theory, assumptions, guesses, predictions, and belief. Without those underlying supports, there could never be progress in science, and there would be no discovery or innovation.

The New Webster Encyclopedic Dictionary of the English Language (Thatcher and McQueen, 1984) defines a theory as follows:

> A supposition explaining something; a doctrine or scheme of things resting merely on speculation; hypothesis; plan or system suggested; an exposition of the general or abstract principles of any science (the *theory* of music or of medicine); the science or rules of an art, as distinguished from the practice; a philosophical explanation of phenomena; a connected arrangement of

facts according to their bearing on some real or hypothetical law or laws. (pp. 368-369)

It is not a criticism or limitation of a theory that it is based on assumptions, logic, and belief. The purpose of theory is to stimulate ways of seeing and investigations that would otherwise not be undertaken. In this book, I emphasize the environmental etiology of the dissociative subtype of schizophrenia because that is the territory opened up by the theory. Human beings could not dissociate without genes any more than they could sing, brush their teeth, get cancer, be born, procreate, or even exist.

This does not mean, however, that there is a gene for brushing teeth. It does not follow from the fact that all behavior, all mental states, and all symptoms depend on the genome that a given mental state with its attendant behavior and symptoms, such as schizophrenia, has a specific genotype. It may, or it may not—determining which is the case is an empirical problem.

Theories have a cultural and historical context and do not occur in a vacuum. At the beginning of the second millennium, the pendulum in psychiatry has swung too far toward endogenous biomedical models of serious mental illness. The theory of a dissociative subtype of schizophrenia is designed to correct the position of the pendulum— its natural tendency is therefore to overcorrect in the direction of environmental and psychosocial factors in the etiology of schizophrenia. Given the current ideological climate in psychiatry and North American culture, however, the pendulum has considerable room before we reach the point of overcorrection.

The purpose of this chapter is not to prove anything or review the evidence; simply I provide an outline of my thinking about genes and environment in psychiatry. The theory of dissociative schizophrenia is built on clinical experience and clinical research data, but its explication requires some attention to the possible relationships between genotype and phenotype in psychiatry.

A MODEL OF GENE-ENVIRONMENT INTERACTION

I propose six possible combinations of genes, environment, and phenotype for the dissociative subtype of schizophrenia, as there are for any psychiatric disorder; these are depicted in Table 1.1. Table 1.1 is an oversimplification for reasons I address later.

TABLE 1.1. Six possible combinations of genes, environment, and phenotype in the dissociative subtype of schizophrenia

	I*	II	III	IV	V	VI
Genotype	+	+	+	−	−	−
Environment	+	−	−	+	+	−
Phenotype	+	+	−	+	−	−

* The roman numerals designate six possible combinations of genes, environment, and phenotype

+ indicates "present"

− indicates "absent"

The environment is the entire universe minus the genome. Intracellular space is part of the environment, as are all events and structures inside the body not including DNA. Environmental causes of dissociative schizophrenia could include viruses, industrial pollutants, closed head injury, street drugs, chronic childhood abuse and neglect, natural or artificial radiation, dietary deficiencies, impaired cerebral circulation, autoimmune encephalitis, prolonged sensory deprivation and isolation, paraneoplastic syndromes, intrauterine infections, and countless other influences.

This list illustrates the many possible environmental causes of schizophrenia. Whether any of these potential causes actually makes an etiological contribution in schizophrenia is an empirical question. I don't address that question here because my purpose in this chapter is to review principles, not evidence.

Table 1.1, as mentioned, is an oversimplification for several reasons. Environmental and genetic causes of schizophrenia are either present or absent in Table 1.1, as is the phenotype. In reality, no doubt all three can be present in varying degrees, resulting in clinical and subclinical syndromes of varying severity.

Table 1.1 has another limitation. Both the genome and the environment can be actively toxic and activate the phenotype, or can be actively healing, soothing, restorative, suppressive, or capable of repair. In the environment, healing, soothing, restorative, and protective factors could include adequate oversight of industry by the Environmental Protection Agency, regulation of radiation exposure, a stable, healthy grandparent, a sound economy, psychotherapy, antipsychotic medication, social services interventions, and the availability of vaccines for infectious diseases. In the genome, regulatory and suppressor genes could protect against abnormal genes, toxic input from the environment, or both.

I assume that the psychosocial environment can both activate and deactivate the phenotype of dissociative schizophrenia, and I assume it can do so in both the presence and the absence of the genotype. I assume that the poorest prognoses and the greatest treatment resistance are associated with the highest number of abnormal genes, the greatest degree of penetration of those genes, and the absence of effective suppressor genes, combined with the presence of toxic environmental input and a deficit of positive environmental input.

I assume that the best prognosis and the greatest degree of treatability occur in cases caused by the psychosocial environment in the absence of the genotype. A more adequate inventory of the possible combinations of genome, environment, and phenotype is presented in Table 1.2.

TABLE 1.2. Thirty-two possible combinations of genes, environment, and phenotype in the dissociative subtype of schizophrenia

	1	2	3	4	5	6	7	8	9	10	11	12	13	14	15	16
NG	+	+	+	+	+	+	+	+	−	−	+	+	+	+	+	+
PG	+	+	+	+	+	+	−	−	+	+	+	+	−	−	−	−
NE	+	+	+	+	−	−	+	+	+	+	−	−	+	+	−	−
PE	+	+	−	−	+	+	+	+	+	+	−	−	−	−	+	+
Ph	+	−	+	−	+	−	+	−	+	−	+	−	+	−	+	−

	17	18	19	20	21	22	23	24	25	26	27	28	29	30	31	32
NG	−	−	−	−	−	−	+	+	−	−	−	−	−	−	−	−
PG	−	−	+	+	+	+	−	−	+	+	−	−	−	−	−	−
NE	+	+	−	−	+	+	−	−	−	−	+	+	−	−	−	−
PE	+	+	+	+	−	−	−	−	−	−	−	−	+	+	−	−
Ph	+	−	+	+	+	−	+	−	+	−	+	−	+	−	+	−

Note: NG = normal genotype; PG = pathological genotype; NE = normal environment; PE = pathological environment; Ph = phenotype

Table 1.2 better approximates reality than does Table 1.1, but it too is an oversimplification, because all four etiological factors and the phenotype can be present to varying degrees; they are continuous rather than dichotomous variables. The effect of the presence or absence of any one of the four variables can be compounded, counteracted, or overridden by the others, depending on which combinations of variables are under consideration. To add another order of complexity, there are many different genes and many different environmental inputs within the cells in Table 1.2, all varying in a continuous fashion.

One purpose of this chapter is to dispel concerns that the theory of a dissociative subtype of schizophrenia is based on a naive or linear model of gene-environment interaction. The theory is primarily clinical in nature. I am not a geneticist, nor do I perform or supervise biological laboratory experiments. My goal is to stimulate a new way of classifying and treating individuals currently receiving treatment for schizophrenia. To achieve that goal, my theory must take genotype and phenotype interactions into account; my focus, however, is on clinical research and treatment that cannot arise from the endogenous biological disease model of schizophrenia.

IMPLICATIONS OF MONOZYGOTIC TWIN DATA

Because the concordance rate for schizophrenia in monozygotic (MZ) twins is under 50 percent (Gottesman, 1991; Sanders and Gejman, 2001; Torrey et al., 1994), at least one of the following three propositions must be true:

1. The environment can activate the genotype to produce the phenotype.
2. The environment can suppress the genotype, so that the phenotype does not occur.
3. The environment can produce the phenotype in the absence of the genotype.

A fourth logical possibility is conceptually trivial but could apply to an unaffected MZ twin in a pair discordant for schizophrenia:

4. The environment can fail to produce the phenotype in the absence of the genotype.

For concordance studies in MZ twins to be relevant, one must assume that MZ twins are genetically identical. Given the base rate of random noise and mutation in any biological system as complex as the genome, this assumption could be challenged; however, I assume that, for practical purposes, MZ twins are genetically identical. This assumption is supported by the 100 percent concordance rate in MZ twins seen in simple Mendelian disorders (see Table 4.1).

MZ twin pairs discordant for schizophrenia are more common than MZ twins concordant for schizophrenia (Gottesman, 1991; Sanders and Gejman, 2001; Torrey et al., 1994). In a discordant twin pair, only two possibilities exist: (a) both twins have the genotype for schizophrenia or (b) both twins do not have the genotype. For any discordant MZ twin pair, one is forced to accept no less than one of three conclusions: (1) if both twins have the genotype, the environment has activated it in the affected twin; (2) if both twins have the genotype, the environment has suppressed it in the unaffected twin; or (3) if both twins do not have the genotype, the environment has caused the phenotype in the affected twin.

On logical grounds, then, everyone must accept at least one of the major postulates of Table 1.2. It is arbitrary which of the two possibilities one chooses to accept for condition (a), because acceptance of one leads inevitably to the conclusion that the other also occurs: if the environment can activate a gene, then it can suppress it, and vice versa. The final outcome of the analysis, then, is that one must accept no less than three of the four logical possibilities (the fourth possibility, absence of the phenotype in the absence of the genotype, is logically trivial). The only one that is subject to controversy or debate is the third possibility, production of the phenotype in the absence of the genotype.

The possibility of a schizophrenic phenotype in the absence of a genotype is not a new or radical idea. It was proposed by Bleuler (1950 [1911] p. 340) when he asked, "Is there a schizophrenia without any hereditary *Anlage?* Probably."

Although the possibility of an environmentally induced form of schizophrenia was acknowledged by Meyer (1911) and Bleuler (1950 [1911]), the search for psychosocial causes of schizophrenia receives very little, if any, funding in psychiatry today. In the absence of a defined and scientifically demonstrated genotype for schizophrenia, the proposition that the genotype must always be present for the phenotype to be manifest is an untestable hypothesis. No identified genotype has yet been identified that can be present or absent.

One could also disagree about whether activation and suppression of the schizophrenic genotype by the environment are limited to the physical environment or include the psychosocial. However, the monozygotic twin concordance data compel everyone to accept the majority of the postulates in Table 1.2.

One purpose of this chapter is to demonstrate that the biopsychosocial assumptions underlying the theory of a dissociative subtype of schizophrenia are consistent with basic logic, the existing data on genes and environment in schizophrenia, and the thinking of leading authorities such as Bleuler (1950 [1911]) and Meyer (1911 [1950]). The only postulate which is potentially controversial in contemporary psychiatry is the proposition that the environment can produce the phenotype in the absence of the genotype.

I discuss this postulate and the genetic model of schizophrenia further in Chapter 4.

THE TRIANGLE OF RECOVERY

I approach both the etiology and the treatment of dissociative schizophrenia in terms of a triangle of recovery. In a truly biopsychosocial model of psychopathology, I believe, one must speak of nature *with* nurture, rather than nature *versus* nurture. Neither the genome nor the environment can function or have meaning without the other. Without an environment, the gene for cystic fibrosis would be an inert string of A-T and G-C base pairs—it would have no biological function and would not be a gene. Conversely, in the absence of the necessary genes, one could not use a toothbrush. Everything in life requires genes somehow to some degree, including the dissociative subtype of schizophrenia. Equally, everything in life requires an environment. Transported to a world without water and oxygen, the human genome could not function. It would not be a genome.

The triangle of recovery has a third corner, the decision-making executive self, which is a testable scientific hypothesis (see Figure 1.1). A human being, I believe, is the product of the interaction of the

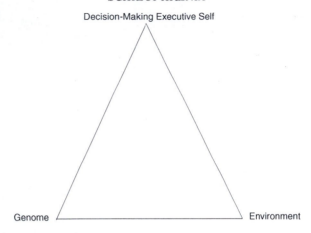

FIGURE 1.1. The triangle of recovery

three corners of this triangle. Each corner has input within limits; no one corner controls or determines all of human behavior. I cannot decide to become a Chinese woman, but I can decide to learn Mandarin Chinese. An alcoholic can decide to become sober. I am the product of my environment, culture, and history, but I can make decisions, including, if I have an addiction or a mental disorder, the commitment to recovery and the work of therapy. I propose that it is possible for psychotherapy to result in long-term, stable remission of the dissociative subtype of schizophrenia. I assume that no corner of the triangle can be reduced to either of the other two.

Although it is housed in the cerebral cortex, the decision-making executive self has spiritual properties that I do not discuss further in this book. That analysis is reserved for future works. Here I pose the question, "How could the existence of the decision-making executive self be demonstrated scientifically?"

First, we must examine the proposition that the self is "housed in the cerebral cortex." This is reductionist language and it violates our current knowledge of physics. The mind cannot be reduced to Newtonian space because matter cannot be reduced to Newtonian space. The mind cannot be accounted for by receptors, transmitters, axonal transport, and other machinery at the biochemical level of the brain because biochemistry can be reduced to physics. Physics provides amore fundamental level of explanation than does biochemistry.

I assume that the decision-making executive self is not located in Newtonian space. It exists at the quantum mechanical level. What happens when the self makes a commitment to recovery from alcoholism, the dissociative subtype of schizophrenia, or any disorder? I assume that an event occurs at the quantum mechanical or subtle energy level of the brain-mind field. This event cannot be caused by Newtonian forces and cannot be explained in terms of three-dimensional space.

A change occurs in the most subtle energy level of the mind. This change then affects the electromagnetic environment of the brain through a trickle-down effect. The electromagnetic environment of the brain-mind field shifts. This shift can be measured as electroencephalogram (EEG) output, although our current technology cannot monitor the most subtle levels of the field. The changes in electromagnetic energy alter the environment of the brain at the biochemical level. This in turn affects the DNA and RNA of brain cells, axonal ions, and other biochemical machinery within the cells. Ultimately, neurotransmission is modulated and the professional monitoring treatment outcome observes new behaviors, feelings, perceptions, and cognitions.

All of this is speculation. However, in a psychotherapy outcome study, researchers could obtain baseline measures using a variety of EEG and brain-imaging technologies. They could then mark the point of serious commitment to recovery on the study timeline. Measures of successful treatment outcome would include reduced psychiatric symptoms, increased psychosocial function, and repaired or normalized central nervous system structure and function. These changes would not occur in control and comparison groups who had not made the commitment to recovery or had not done the work of therapy.

I am not suggesting that one can decide not to have schizophrenia and instantly be well. The commitment to recovery initiates a long, arduous process that results in brain self-repair over an extended period of time. The purpose of the theory of dissociative schizophrenia is to identify a subgroup in which this outcome is more likely. The theory states that effective psychotherapy of the nondissociative sub-types is less likely but not impossible.

I expand on these themes in the final section of this book, and they are developed in preliminary fashion *The Trauma Model: A Solution to the Problem of Comorbidity in Psychiatry* (Ross, 2000b).

The brain can be understood as a harmonics generator. We know this to be a fact because of EEG technology. The brain generates different electromagnetic energy waves. Similar to the harmonics in a concert hall, the initial waves must interact with one another to produce harmonics. The harmonics must interact to produce another, more subtle level of waves, and this process must occur through a series of levels until the signals are attenuated to an undetectable level. The mind, I propose, is the subtle harmonic level of this field.

The proposed psychotherapy outcome study would demonstrate that causality can run from the top of the brain-mind field down to the level of biochemical function and anatomical change. The change could include neuronal and dendritic regeneration and growth in the hippocampus, for instance. Whatever the specific biological outcome measures, the principle of the model is that causality can run in all possible directions in the system. Countless feedback loops, regulatory mechanisms, and interactions occur within the system.

This model of the brain-mind field permits the activation of the schizophrenia phenotype by the psychosocial environment and also by the genome. If a model of this type is not permitted, then the psychosocial origins of the dissociative subtype of schizophrenia are not possible. My purpose here is not to provide evidence for any of the details used to illustrate the principles of the theory. I am simply describing the type of mind-body model that must be true for the theory of a dissociative subtype of schizophrenia to be valid.

The proposition that the mind can be reduced to brain structures and biochemistry is, in my view, unscientific. This has been true since the twentieth century when Newtonian reductionism was supplanted by quantum mechanics and relativity theory. Adequate models of mental illness in the twenty-first century cannot be based on the logic or processes of nineteenth-century physics.

The dissociative subtype of schizophrenia is simultaneously a biological, psychological, social, and spiritual problem. Therapeutic interventions can be made at any and all of these levels. Intervention at any level can have an impact at any other level. Medications alter the mind and psychotherapy alters the brain. These assumptions are included here to lay the foundation for subsequent arguments in favor of the existence of a dissociative subtype of schizophrenia.

A core postulate of my theory is the activation of the genome by the psychosocial environment. The strands of DNA activated by psychological trauma could be normal, abnormal, or a mixture of both. This postulate is endorsed by Sapolsky in a review of the possibilities for gene therapy of psychiatric disorders. Sapolsky (2003) states that "the critical concept that must be emphasized endlessly is that the biology of psychiatric disorders is not about inevitability but is instead about vulnerability and propensity. It is only in certain environments that the disease is likely to emerge" (p. 214).

Sapolsky (2003) reviews the activation of cortisol by stress, which in turn activates strands of DNA called cortisol-responsive elements. Future gene therapy for stress-induced depression, Sapolsky says, could involve manipulation of strands of DNA involved in the response to stress-induced increases in cortisol. The genetic vulnerability to depression, in such a model, need not be a "gene for depression" as such, and the strands of DNA involved need not be abnormal. Sapolsky's model is the same as the one I am proposing here, in that it allows the production of DSM-IV-TR disorders by the interaction of psychological trauma with the normal genome.

Chapter 2

Characteristics of the Dissociative Subtype of Schizophrenia

The DSM-IV-TR (American Psychiatric Association, 2000) describes three subtypes of schizophrenia: paranoid, catatonic, and disorganized. These correspond to Bleuler's (1950 [1911]) subtypes of paranoid, catatonic, and hebephrenic. Bleuler's fourth subtype of simple schizophrenia corresponds to the Axis II, Cluster A diagnoses of paranoid, schizoid, and schizotypal personality disorders.

It is not likely that early in the twenty-first century the field of psychiatry has exhaustively cataloged all the valid and reliable subtypes of schizophrenia. Bleuler (1950 [1911]) spoke of the *group of schizophrenias* in the original 1911 German edition of his classic text, and virtually all authorities and textbooks since have agreed that the clinical syndrome of schizophrenia encompasses numerous different diseases and etiological pathways. The postulate of a dissociative subtype of schizophrenia is consistent with accepted thinking in the field concerning the existence of unrecognized subtypes of schizophrenia.

This chapter outlines the basic characteristics of the dissociative subtype of schizophrenia. The evidence for the subtype is the focus of the remainder of the book.

THE SPECTRUM FROM NONDISSOCIATIVE SUBTYPES OF SCHIZOPHRENIA TO DISSOCIATIVE IDENTITY DISORDER

When I first coined the term *dissociative subtype of schizophrenia* in the mid-1990s, I organized it along the continuum shown in Figure 2.1. I originally devised this spectrum to differentiate the dissociative subtype of schizophrenia from nondissociative schizophrenia at the

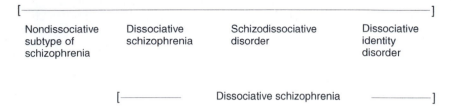

FIGURE 2.1. The spectrum of a dissociative subtype of schizophrenia

left end, and from dissociative identity disorder (DID, multiple personality disorder) at the right end. The nondissociative subtypes of schizophrenia are the paranoid, catatonic, and undifferentiated forms described in Bleuler (1950 [1911]) and in the DSM-IV-TR. I proposed the existence of a disorder intermediate between DID and dissociative schizophrenia, analogous to schizoaffective disorder, which is intermediate between schizophrenia and mood disorders. I called this entity *schizodissociative disorder.*

The less complex dissociative disorders (dissociative amnesia, dissociative fugue, and depersonalization disorder) could not be subsumed under dissociative schizophrenia. They are not complex, severe, or chronic enough. However, chronic, complex forms of dissociative disorder not otherwise specified (DDNOS) could be included within dissociative schizophrenia since they are often slightly milder variants of DID.

Since the mid-1990s, as discussed in the preface, I have considered an alternative approach: it would be possible, in principle, to include all disorders to the right of nondissociative subtypes of schizophrenia within the single category of dissociative schizophrenia. The basic problem is not simply one of comorbidity and differential diagnosis. The DSM-IV-TR positive symptom criteria for schizophrenia are more characteristic of DID than of schizophrenia. The core features of DID are found in Bleuler's schizophrenia and the core features of schizophrenia are found in the DSM-IV-TR DID criteria. Because of the way the two disorders are defined in the DSM-IV-TR and the clinical and research literatures, they cannot be separated into two discrete categories. They are too much and too often the same thing.

Incorporating DID as a subtype of schizophrenia would solve the problem of differential diagnosis but would create other problems.

For instance, what would be the relationship between dissociative schizophrenia, the other diagnoses remaining in the dissociative disorders section of the DSM, and post-traumatic stress disorder (PTSD)?

Practical Problems

Since the turn of the millennium, I have increasingly favored classifying all cases to the right of the nondissociative subtypes within the single category of dissociative schizophrenia. This approach would have both pros and cons. If DID was reclassified as a subtype of schizophrenia, then the possibility of a traumatic form of schizophrenia treatable with psychotherapy would arise. This would improve the prognosis for schizophrenia as a whole and provide a valid subtype of schizophrenia in which the phenotype can occur with and without the genotype. The risk for the dissociative subtype of schizophrenia would be especially elevated in cells three, seven, thirteen, fourteen and twenty-seven in Table 1.2.

The risk of reclassifying DID as a subtype of schizophrenia is that psychotherapy for DID might disappear on the grounds that schizophrenia cannot be treated with psychotherapy. In the current medicolegal environment, one can withhold neuroleptics and provide psychotherapy for DID with much less risk to the treating professional than if the same person is given a diagnosis of schizophrenia.

Reclassifying DID as a subtype of schizophrenia might result in affected individuals receiving much larger amounts of antipsychotic medication. This would increase their risk for tardive dyskinesia, neuroleptic malignant syndrome, drug-induced diabetes and weight gain, sedation, and other side effects and complications. It might increase the likelihood of affected individuals perceiving themselves as untreatable with psychotherapy, which in turn would increase the likelihood of their dropping out of therapy. A reclassification might change the type of family therapy provided, shifting it away from a therapeutic systems orientation to a more supportive and educational mode.

Also, negative stereotypes about schizophrenia might be projected onto people with DID if they were reclassified as having a form of schizophrenia. These stereotypes could include the belief that people with schizophrenia are "crazy," dangerous, unpredictable, dirty, untreatable, or unemployable. The legal status of people with DID might change as well—they might be more eligible for the insanity defense, for instance, or for disability, pensions, and government services.

Although I recognize that the dissociative subtype of schizophrenia could have numerous political, legal, and sociological implications, I do not discuss them further in this book. My focus here is on defining a clinical problem, achieving its recognition, and proposing a solution. If the dissociative subtype of schizophrenia is recognized in the field, it will be important to debate and think about its possible social ramifications.

At present, DID and its treatment are marginalized within academic psychiatry and there is little serious psychotherapy for schizophrenia, beyond supportive and educational interventions. For this to change, either DID must be accepted or a trauma pathway to schizophrenia must be accepted. There is resistance to both options within academic psychiatry. Therefore, from a practical perspective, it is unclear which option to endorse. Scientifically, I favor including all disorders to the right of nondissociative subtypes of schizophrenia within the single category of dissociative schizophrenia.

I would expect my DID patients to be bewildered by having their diagnoses changed to dissociative schizophrenia until the new nomenclature was explained to them. If such a change was incorporated in a future edition of DSM, I would remind the patients that schizophrenia and DID are only words and that many individuals made the transition from multiple personality disorder to DID quite smoothly in 1994 with the publication of the DSM-IV (American Psychiatric Association, 1994).

Properties

The dissociative subtype of schizophrenia has the properties shown in Box 2.1. For the dissociative subtype of schizophrenia to be valid, each of these properties must be operationalized and subjected to research with valid and reliable measures. Some of this work has been done, but by no means all.

Dissociative schizophrenia is well described in the 1950 English translation of Bleuler's classic 1911 text, *Dementia Praecox or the Group of Schizophrenias.* Advances in the clinical, research, and psychometric

---

**BOX 2.1. Properties of the dissociative subtype
of schizophrenia**

————————————————————————————————➤

Moving right on the spectrum, one encounters:

- Fewer negative symptoms of schizophrenia
- More positive symptoms of schizophrenia
- Less thought disorder
- More comorbidity on Axis I and Axis II (including more dissociative disorders and post-traumatic stress disorder
- More psychobiology of trauma
- Less psychobiology of endogenous psychosis
- More response to psychotherapy
- Less response to neuroleptic medication
- Increased frequency of oculogyric crises and dystonic reactions to medication
- More structure and defined ego states
- More ability of voices to engage in rational conversation
- More ability of voices to take executive control
- Higher scores on measures of dissociation
- Higher scores on measures of hypnotizability
- More severe and chronic childhood trauma
- More dissociative schizophrenia in relatives
- Less nondissociative schizophrenia in relatives
- Better prognosis

---

literature on dissociation in the past twenty years (see Chapter 9) make it possible to operationalize the dissociative subtype of schizophrenia, but most of its properties are explicit in Bleuler's original description. Cases of dissociative schizophrenia exist in the recent psychiatric literature as well, and examples are presented in Chapter 12, with he caveat that definitive diagnoses cannot be made from written case summaries.

PART II:
PSYCHOSIS AND SCHIZOPHRENIA

Chapter 3

Definitions of Psychosis
and Schizophrenia

The term *psychosis* has a variety of different meanings. Operationalized definitions are available in standardized self-report and interviewer-administered measures reviewed by Pincus et al. (2000). These include the Brief Psychiatric Rating Scale (BPRS) (Overall and Gorham, 1988), the Scale for Assessment of Negative Symptoms (SANS) (Andreasen, 1983), the Scale for Assessment of Positive Symptoms (SAPS) (Andreasen, 1984), and the Positive and Negative Syndrome Scale (PANSS) (Kay, Opler, and Fiszbein, 1994), all of which have good psychometric properties.

The clinical meaning of psychosis is more elusive than the meaning used in the BPRS, SAPS, SANS, and PANSS, and varies by continent, time period, and theoretical orientation of the person using the term. Currently, in clinical practice in North America, *psychotic* means that the person has a biomedical brain disease or a chemical imbalance, requires medication, and cannot be treated with psychotherapy. *Neurotic,* in contrast, means that the person has a chronic or acute life adjustment problem and may be treated with psychotherapy and/or medication.

Often, psychotic means severe mental illness and neurotic means mild. The symptoms that go along with psychosis include hallucinations, delusions, thought disorder, disorganization, agitation, catatonia, and bizarre speech or behavior. Psychosis includes less insight and reduced social and occupational function. All of these criteria are a matter of degree, however, and do not distinguish between mild psychosis and severe neurosis.

The problem of the overlap versus the difference between psychosis and neurosis is unsolved, although both terms are often used as if their meanings are clear. In this book I adhere to the DSM-IV-TR definitions of psychosis and schizophrenia.

DSM-IV-TR DEFINITION OF PSYCHOSIS

The ambiguity inherent in the various definitions of psychosis is well described in the DSM-IV-TR:

> The term *psychotic* has historically received a number of different definitions, none of which have received universal acceptance. The narrowest definition of *psychotic* is restricted to delusions or prominent hallucinations, with the hallucinations occurring in the absence of insight into their pathological nature. A slightly less restrictive definition would also include prominent hallucinations that the individual realizes are hallucinatory experiences. Broader still is a definition that also includes other positive symptoms of Schizophrenia (i.e., disorganized speech, grossly disorganized or catatonic behavior). Unlike these definitions based on symptoms, the definition used in earlier classifications (e.g., DSM-II and ICD-9) was probably far too inclusive and focused on the severity of functional impairment. In that context, a mental disorder was termed "psychotic" if it resulted in "impairment that grossly interferes with the capacity to meet ordinary demands of life." The term has also previously been defined as a "loss of ego boundaries" or a "gross impairment in reality testing."
>
> In this manual, the term *psychotic* refers to the presence of certain symptoms. However, the specific constellation of symptoms to which the term refers varies to some extent across the diagnostic categories. In Schizophrenia, Schizophreniform Disorder, Schizoaffective Disorder, and Brief Psychotic Disorder, the term *psychotic* refers to delusions, any prominent hallucinations, disorganized speech, or disorganized or catatonic behavior. In Psychotic Disorder Due to a General Medical Condition and in Substance-Induced Psychotic Disorder, *psychotic* refers to delusions or only those hallucinations that are not accompanied by insight. Finally, in Delusional Disorder and Shared Psychotic Disorder, *psychotic* is equivalent to delusional. (Reprinted

with permission from the *Diagnostic and Statistical Manual of Mental Disorders,* Text Revision, pp. 297-298. Copyright 2000. American Psychiatric Association.)

Many of these psychotic symptoms are more characteristic of nineteenth-century hysteria and contemporary DID than they are of DSM-IV-TR schizophrenia. For instance, auditory hallucinations and other Schneiderian symptoms are more common in DID than they are in schizophrenia (see Chapters 9, 10, and 11 for data and further discussion). Nevertheless, since they are the accepted and working definitions of psychosis in contemporary psychiatry, I adhere to them.

DSM-IV-TR TEXT AND CRITERIA FOR SCHIZOPHRENIA

Schizophrenia is a subset of psychosis. Psychotic symptoms can have numerous causes and can occur in a variety of DSM-IV-TR categories. However, schizophrenia cannot occur without psychosis.

The DSM-IV-TR criteria for schizophrenia pose a major problem for the field. Schizophrenia is widely regarded as the most severe mental illness. It is not plausible, biologically or medically, that a severe, complex, and heterogeneous disease can be diagnosed based on a single positive symptom, as allowed by DSM-IV-TR.

The DSM-IV-TR diagnostic Criterion A for schizophrenia is shown in Box 3.1. Criterion B is a requirement for deterioration in social or occupational function; Criterion C is a requirement for a duration of six months; and Criteria D, E, and F discuss the relationship between schizophrenia and other disorders.

Schizophrenia is the equivalent of *cough disorder* or *fever disorder.* The idea that fever could be a unitary biomedical disease with a specific genetic cause is implausible. It would never be advanced in general medicine, yet similar logic is endorsed by the American Psychiatric Association in the DSM-IV-TR criteria for schizophrenia. Auditory hallucinations, including two or more voices commenting on each other, are a characteristic symptom of DID. They are more common in DID than in schizophrenia. Yet DID is regarded as a neurotic disorder. Auditory hallucinations can also occur in mania, delirium,

---

BOX 3.1. DSM-IV-TR diagnostic criteria for schizophrenia

A. Characteristic symptoms: Two (or more) of the following, each present for a significant portion of time during a one-month period (or less if successfully treated):
    (1) delusions
    (2) hallucinations
    (3) disorganized speech (e.g., frequent derailment or incoherence)
    (4) grossly disorganized or catatonic behavior
    (5) negative symptoms, i.e., affective flattening, alogia, or avolition

Note: Only one Criterion A symptom is required if delusions are bizarre or hallucinations consist of a voice keeping up a running commentary on the person's behavior or thoughts, or two or more voices commenting on each other.

Source: Reprinted by permission from the *Diagnostic and Statistical Manual of Mental Disorders,* Fourth Edition, Text Revision, p. 312. Copyright 2000 American Psychiatric Association.

---

organic brain syndromes, and members of the general population with no measurable psychopathology or dysfunction (Honig et al., 1998).

Because the DSM-IV-TR criteria provide the accepted and working definition of schizophrenia in psychiatry, I adhere to them in this book. There is no other "schizophrenia" to talk about because, at present, the only way to determine that a person has schizophrenia is if he or she meets DSM-IV-TR criteria for the disorder. A person has nondissociative schizophrenia if he or she meets criteria for the paranoid, catatonic, or undifferentiated subtypes.

In this book I do not discuss the problem of differential diagnosis between the paranoid, catatonic, and undifferentiated forms of schizophrenia. It is clear that these subtypes are not stable and that individuals can drift back and forth between them over time. I treat them as a single group. I do not plan to study the overlap or degree of difference between the dissociative and nondissociative subtypes of schizophrenia until an operationalized definition of the dissociative subtype has been accepted in the field. However, I assume that such overlap will be found and that it will be reduced by refinement of subtype criteria based on the results of empirical studies. The overlap between schizophrenia and dissociative identity disorder is discussed at length in Chapter 11.

Chapter 4

The Genetic Model of Schizophrenia

The data on twin concordance rates for schizophrenia demonstrate conclusively that the genome is a minor contributor to the disorder. Torrey (1992) and Torrey et al. (1994) summarized the results of eight studies they considered sufficiently rigorous for analysis. They found that overall concordance in 341 pairs of MZ twins was 28 percent compared to 6 percent in 587 pairs of dizygotic (DZ) twins. When the authors restricted the analysis to the three studies they considered most rigorous (Fischer, 1973; Kringlen, 1967; Tienari, 1963), concordance in 86 monozygotic twin pairs was 26 percent, while in 173 dizygotic twin pairs it was 8 percent.

The difference between MZ and DZ twins in concordance for schizophrenia is statistically significant. However, in identical twins concordance is under 30 percent. That is the primary fact that should be the focus of discussion, theory, and funding for research on the causes of schizophrenia.

Sanders and Gejman (2001) concurred with this summary of the literature in a more recent review. They stated that the ratio of MZ:DZ concordance for schizophrenia is in the range of 3:1 to 4:1. Despite these data on twin concordance, however, and despite the fact that such findings have been available in the literature for four decades, it is still widely believed that schizophrenia is a predominantly genetic disorder.

For instance, Kendler (1998) stated, in accepting the Dean Award for his lifetime work on schizophrenia from the American College of Psychiatrists, "Most if not all the reason why schizophrenia runs in families is due to shared genes and not shared environment." In the same acceptance speech, he presented his own data on 16,000 twin pairs in which concordance for schizophrenia in MZ twins was 31 percent.

Similarly, Cannon et al. (1998), in their study of concordance in a large sample of Finnish twins, found an MZ concordance rate of 45 percent. They concluded from their data that 83 percent of the variance was accounted for by genetic factors. The Cannon et al. (1998) statistical procedure might imply that the causation of schizophrenia is predominantly genetic, but it isn't, and can't be, because of the low concordance rate.

The belief that schizophrenia is predominantly genetic has been widely accepted among patient support groups and the general population. It can be found on a variety of Web pages. This information is reviewed in Chapter 11.

THE GENOME AS A MINOR CONTRIBUTOR TO THE CAUSES OF SCHIZOPHRENIA

Table 4.1 places the concordance rate for schizophrenia in MZ twins in context. Some normal human traits and some diseases are purely genetic. The risk for developing cystic fibrosis is not affected by the environment, although prognosis and outcome are highly responsive to environmental variables including antibiotics, respiratory

TABLE 4.1. Concordance rates in monozygotic twins

Variable	Concordance rate (%)
Race	100
Eye color	100
Gender	100
Huntington's chorea	100
Cystic fibrosis	100
Tay-Sachs disease	100
Epilepsy	61
Mental retardation	60
Schizophrenia	28
Parkinson's disease	27

Source: Adapted from Torrey et al., 1994.

therapy, enzyme replacement, the economics of the health care system, and the psychological health and motivation of the parents to provide optimal care.

Other disorders such as epilepsy and mental retardation are intermediate in their etiology. Concordance in MZ twins for these disorders is above 50 percent but, on the other hand, is substantially less than 100 percent. It is clear that both the genome and the environment are major players in the etiology of epilepsy and mental retardation.

In disorders such as schizophrenia and Parkinson's disease, the genome is a minor contributor. In these two disorders, there is a genetic contribution to etiology because MZ concordance is greater than DZ concordance, but it is outweighed by the effects of the environment.

Based on the MZ concordance rate of 28 percent, we can conclude that schizophrenia is less than one-third genetic. The true genetic concordance is likely less than 28 percent because the equal environments assumption probably does not hold for schizophrenia. According to the equal environments assumption, the psychosocial environment treats MZ twins the same to the same degree that it treats DZ twins the same. This is not the case, however.

Common experience and a large social science literature prove that MZ twins are treated the same more often than DZ twins are. They more often have first names that start with the same letter, are in the same classrooms, wear matching clothes, have the same friends, sleep in the same bedrooms, and share the same activities, and they are mistaken for each other more often (Pam et al., 1996).

Because the environments of MZ twins are more equal than the environments of DZ twins, some of the increased concordance for schizophrenia in MZ twins could be due to the environment. The effect of this greater degree of shared environment is unlikely to be less than 3 percent; therefore one can conclude that the true genetic concordance for schizophrenia in MZ twins is likely less than 25 percent. Even if this argument is rejected, MZ twin concordance for schizophrenia is definitely in the range of 28 to 35 percent, while DZ concordance is about 10 percent. The environment is definitely a greater contributor to etiology than the genome, although it is equally true that the genome does make a contribution.

The fact that the environment treats MZ twins the same more than it treats DZ twins the same doesn't mean it always treats them exactly the same—if it did, MZ concordance would be 100 percent. The basic premise of my theory is that differential environmental input causes MZ twin concordance to be only 28 percent. Indeed, there is no other logical or scientific possibility.

Let me reiterate: schizophrenia has a genetic component. This fact is proven by the difference between MZ and DZ twin concordance rates. However, the data are clear and unequivocal: the causes of schizophrenia are more environmental than genetic. The environmental causes of schizophrenia could include biological variables such as intrauterine infections and birth injuries (Torrey et al., 1994), as discussed in Chapter 1. A reduced emphasis on genetic causes of schizophrenia would not necessarily mean a reduced emphasis on biology. For instance, the role of biology in schizophrenia could increase if the psychobiology of trauma was taken seriously in the schizophrenia field.

Studies of the effects of adoption on children born to a schizophrenic parent (Pam, 1995) show that adoption out of a schizophrenic family reduces the risk for developing schizophrenia by two-thirds. This reduction is solely attributable to the environment, probably the psychosocial environment. The existing data clearly demonstrate that the environment can suppress expression of the schizophrenia phenotype. To argue otherwise, one would have to propose that the unaffected adopted-out children of schizophrenic parents did not have the genotype for schizophrenia—this argument could not preserve a genetic model of schizophrenia

In addition, schizophrenia does not breed true. First-degree relatives of individuals with schizophrenia have increased rates of schizophrenia and mood disorders. Inversely, first-degree relatives of individuals with mood disorders have increased rates of mood disorders and schizophrenia (Taylor et al., 1993). Both groups of relatives have higher rates of both mood disorders and schizophrenia than the relatives of unaffected controls. As Goff (2002, pp. 3255-3256) states, "Interestingly, a good deal of research suggests that the genetics are not following the diagnostic categories that we have traditionally used clinically."

Stein et al. (2002) concluded from a study of 222 MZ twins and 184 DZ twins that a genetic contribution to PTSD exists, but that it is basically an inherited temperament, not an inherited diagnosis. PTSD-prone individuals, they suggested, inherit a more volatile emotional makeup that results in greater exposure to trauma and greater reactivity to the trauma once it occurs. The genetic predisposition to schizophrenia might interact with the environment in a similar fashion, and it might be a predisposition to a broad range of psychopathology, not just to schizophrenia. The etiological model proposed by Stein et al. (2002) for PTSD is interactive and bidirectional. It allows causality to run both from genome to environment and from environment to genome; I am suggesting that the same logic should be applied to schizophrenia.

From the time of the Danish adoption studies (Kety et al., 1968; Pam, 1995), researchers have had difficulty establishing an increased risk for narrowly defined schizophrenia in the relatives of affected individuals. Often, in order to obtain significant results, investigators have had to broaden the definition of affected relatives to include a variety of spectrum disorders. This strategy provides additional evidence that schizophrenia does not breed true—what breeds true is a spectrum of disorders that encompasses a number of different DSM-IV-TR categories.

The data support the conclusion that the genetic risk is not for specific DSM-IV-TR categories such as schizophrenia but for psychopathology in general. Torrey et al. (1994), for instance, describe pedigrees that include individuals with both schizophrenia and bipolar mood disorder. This finding has been consistent in the literature for four decades, is an everyday aspect of clinical experience and history taking in general psychiatry, and is supported by mathematical models of the genetic overlap between bipolar mood disorder, schizoaffective disorder, and schizophrenia (Cardino et al., 2002).

I propose a modified type of concordance study. Researchers should divide twins into two categories: those with (1) presence of severe psychopathology and (2) absence of severe psychopathology. I predict that concordance for severe psychopathology spanning a broad range of DSM-IV-TR categories is substantially higher than concordance rates for single diagnostic categories. This finding would be consistent with the fact that 90 percent of individuals with schizophrenia do not have a relative with schizophrenia; 70 percent of MZ twins with schizophrenia have an unaffected twin.

In this modified type of concordance study, psychosocial trauma would be a key variable. I predict that severe psychopathology would be most common in individuals with severe trauma. The highest rates of concordance for severe psychopathology would occur in MZ twins concordant for severe trauma. The lowest rates of concordance would occur in DZ twins discordant for trauma. DZ twins concordant for trauma and MZ twins discordant for trauma would have intermediate rates of concordance for severe psychopathology. This design would demonstrate the input of both the genome and the psychosocial environment in the etiology of severe psychopathology.

In one study, 70 percent of adult MZ twins discordant for schizophrenia were indistinguishable as children on variables including neurological status, personality traits, interpersonal function, school function, birth complications, medical history, and head injury (Torrey et al., 1994). No definite conclusion can be drawn from this finding, but it is consistent with schizophrenia caused by being differential environmental input occurring after early childhood. Early childhood trauma may have contributed to schizophrenia among the affected individuals in this study; if it did, its effects were not apparent in the variables measured by Torrey et al. (1994).

In their study of MZ twins discordant for schizophrenia, Torrey et al. (1994) found no significant differences between the twins on minor physical anomalies, birth weights, or left-handedness. The absence of such differences argues against intrauterine events or complications of delivery being causes of the discordance. Torrey et al. (1994) were also unable to demonstrate differential rates of head injury or physical illness in discordant MZ twin pairs.

All of these negative findings point to the psychosocial environment as a possible source of the 72 percent discordance for schizophrenia among MZ twins. The existing data, accumulated over four decades, clearly and consistently demonstrate that schizophrenia is predominantly an environmentally induced disorder. To date, no diagnostically specific biological marker for schizophrenia, including genetic markers, has been found. It is always possible that such a marker exists, but it hasn't yet been demonstrated.

Joober et al. (2002, p. 343) state, "Indeed, it is becoming clear that, as in the field of neuropathology, where a gross neuropathological signature of schizophrenia does not exist, major genes causing schizophrenia do not exist."

I quote these authors because their work in molecular genetics is funded by RGS Genome Inc., the National Alliance for Research on Schizophrenia and Depression, and the Canadian Institutes of Health Research. They are career behavioral geneticists and therefore are highly invested in finding specific genetic underpinnings for schizophrenia. Their conclusion cannot be dismissed as based on ideological hostility to the genetic model of schizophrenia.

MZ twins discordant for schizophrenia are frequently discordant for biological variables of interest, such as increased ventricular volume and decreased volume of the hippocampus and amygdala (Nelson et al., 1998; Szeszko et al., 2002; Torrey et al., 1994). One cause of reduced hippocampal volume in laboratory mammals is high levels of cortisol induced by psychological trauma (Bremner and Marmer, 1998; Bremner et al., 1995; Heim and Nemeroff, 1999; Markowitsch et al., 1998; Read, Perry, et al., 2001; Sapolsky, 2000; Teuchert-Noodt, 2000). Therefore, reduced hippocampal volume and increased ventricular volume are compatible with psychosocial causation of schizophrenia.

Further research is required to determine the causes of such biological findings in schizophrenia; my point here is that the evidence to date is consistent with environmental causes of schizophrenia and does not weigh in favor of genetic causes. A common logical error in psychiatry is to assume that biological findings in the literature to date favor genetic and endogenous biological causes of schizophrenia, which is not true.

In summary, the existing data provide overwhelming, replicated, and conclusive evidence that the genome is a minor contributor to the causes of schizophrenia. The environment is far more important. The difference in concordance rates between MZ and DZ twins is a true, significant finding; however, it is outweighed by the 28 percent concordance rate for schizophrenia in MZ twins. It is scientifically impossible that the causes of DSM-IV-TR schizophrenia are mostly genetic.

EVIDENCE FOR THE TOXIC AND PROTECTIVE EFFECTS OF THE PSYCHOSOCIAL ENVIRONMENT

There are many critiques of studies purporting to have demonstrated a genetic predisposition to schizophrenia (Boyle, 1990; Jay,

2001; Rose, 1991; Ross and Pam, 1995; Turkheimer, 1998) or other adult disorders (Goldberg, 2001). One problem in genetic research is the failure of investigators to study the psychological health of families adopting the offspring of schizophrenic mothers. One of the rare studies of the genetics of schizophrenia that evaluated the families adopting the offspring of schizophrenic mothers found that only 4 percent of those children raised by "healthy" adoptive families were diagnosed as "severe psychotic," compared to 34 percent of the children raised by "disturbed" adoptive families (Tienari, 1991). Among the family dimensions correlated to the children's mental health, at the $p < .0001$ level, were: "expelling relation to offspring" (i.e., ejection) and "conflict between parents and offspring." Tienari concluded that "in healthy rearing families the adoptees have little serious mental illness, whether or not their biological mothers were schizophrenic" (1991, p. 463).

The level of functioning of the adopting families produced an improvement chi-square (measuring the extent to which a variable gives more information, that is, improves the model) of 40.22 ($p < .0001$) while the improvement chi-square of the genetic variable (whether or not the biological mother was schizophrenic) was only 5.78 ($p < .016$). Thus the dysfunction of the family, and the rejection of the child implied thereby, had seven times more explanatory power than genetic predisposition.

All data in which MZ twins discordant for schizophrenia are discordant for structural brain abnormalities presumed to be causally related to the clinical syndrome are conclusive proof of a major environmental contribution (Suddath et al., 1990; Torrey et al., 1994). Families with discordant twin pairs should be studied carefully from a psychosocial perspective because the healing, restorative, or protective effect of the environment on the unaffected twin or, conversely, the toxic effect of the environment on the affected twin could be demonstrated in such families.

I argued previously that the equal environments assumption probably does not hold for MZ/DZ twin studies in schizophrenia. The fact that the environment treats MZ twins the same more than it does DZ twins does not mean it treats MZ twins *exactly* the same. The 28 percent MZ concordance proves two things: the cause of schizophrenia is mostly environmental and the environment treats MZ twins differently to a major degree. If it did not, concordance would be much higher than 28 percent.

For psychological trauma to be relevant in the etiology of schizophrenia, the environment must play a significant role. This postulate is consistent with current multifactorial etiological models of schizophrenia (Tienari and Wynne, 1994). Severe adverse events in childhood might contribute, either independently or in interaction with the effects of genetic risk or perinatal factors (Kunugi, Nanko, and Murray, 2001), to the production of schizophrenia. Once this possibility is considered, variables assumed to be markers of endogenous biological etiology may prove to be, instead, markers of toxic environmental input. For instance, a deficit in performance of smooth pursuit eye movement tasks, usually assumed to be a biological marker of the genetic predisposition to schizophrenia, is significantly related to physical and emotional abuse in childhood (Irwin, Green, and Marsh, 1999). Similarly, reduced hippocampal volume in schizophrenia is attributed to genetic factors and perinatal hypoxia by van Erp et al. (2002), but could be due to psychological trauma in a subset of cases.

The existing data on twin and family studies and on biological variables in schizophrenia provide overwhelming evidence that the disorder is predominantly environmental in its etiology. The likelihood of finding a diagnostically specific genome for schizophrenia, except in a small subset of cases, is minimal because schizophrenia does not breed true. Only one scientific conclusion can be drawn from an MZ twin concordance of 28 percent—it is impossible that schizophrenia is predominantly genetic. It must be predominantly environmental. To reiterate, this does not mean that the genome makes no contribution.

As I have argued repeatedly, the genome appears to contribute a diagnostically nonspecific predisposition to psychopathology in general. This predisposition appears to interact with the environment in a complex bidirectional fashion. Unidirectional genetic causation of specific DSM-IV-TR categories does not seem to occur in nature, except possibly in a small minority of pedigrees.

It is proven that two individuals with the same genome can be discordant for schizophrenia. The reciprocal is also true, in my clinical experience: two individuals with similar family backgrounds and high levels of chronic trauma can be discordant for schizophrenia. In my opinion, except perhaps in a small number of pedigrees, there is no "gene for schizophrenia" to discover in nature. MZ twin concordance is too low; the disorder does not breed true; the DSM-IV-TR Criterion A symptoms are too nonspecific; and there is too much comorbidity for the genetic model of schizophrenia to be correct, except for a small minority of cases. This is true no matter how polygenetic or complex the genetic model of schizophrenia under consideration.

The inherited predisposition, I propose, is to psychopathology in general, not to specific DSM-IV-TR categories. This predisposition is captured better by the concept of temperament than it is by the concept of psychiatric diagnosis.

From a public health perspective, molecular biology approaches to DSM-IV-TR schizophrenia are unlikely to be more fruitful than similar approaches to infectious diseases. It is obvious that some individuals are more hardy than others, in terms of susceptibility to infection, but no gene exists for the common cold, bacterial pneumonia, AIDS, bacterial nephritis, or any other of the common infectious diseases. All of those forms of infection interact with myriad regulatory mechanisms within the human organism, all of which are ultimately encoded in our DNA, but this does not mean that there are specific genetic causes of different, common forms of viral exanthem, pneumonia, or nephritis. We should apply the same medical logic to schizophrenia.

Psychiatry's approach to schizophrenia is in some ways similar to the medical profession's approach to obesity. Flegal et al. (2002) reported that the age-adjusted rate of obesity among American adults in 1999-2000 was 30.5 percent compared to 22.9 percent in 1988-1994. Obesity was defined as a body mass index above 30, based on direct physical examination of 3,601 adult subjects. Ogden et al. (2002) reported the age-adjusted rate of obesity among 4,722 American children. For children ages twelve to nineteen years, the rate was 15.5 percent in 1999-2000 compared to 10.5 percent in 1988-1994; for those ages six to eleven years, it was 15.3 percent compared to 11.3 percent; and for those ages two to five years, it was 10.4 percent compared to 7.2 percent.

There is no possibility that this increase in obesity was due to changes in the underlying biology or genetics of the population. It is 100 percent certain that this increase was driven entirely by the environment. Yet, in a call for papers on obesity research in the same issue of the *Journal of the American Medical Association,* Fontanarosa (2002) wrote,

> Basic science investigations have revealed new knowledge about the complex molecular, genetic, and biological mechanisms of obesity, appetite, and metabolism. . . . Papers describing basic science and translational research investigations that provide novel insights about the underlying pathophysiology of obesity also will receive careful consideration.

Similar to the situation in psychiatry, the role of the psychosocial environment in obesity is recognized in theory by the medical profession. In practice, however, there is a disproportionate investment of resources and intellectual energy in genetics and "underlying pathophysiology." This misallocation of medical resources does not match the relative contributions of genome and culture to obesity in North America.

The proposition that the causes of epidemic obesity in America can be found in an underlying pathophysiology is based on the same biomechanistic model that dominates contemporary psychiatry. Lip service is paid to the environment, but the investment of time, energy, and resources in biological studies far outweighs the actual etiological role of genes and molecules. The balance between nature and nurture in contemporary medicine and psychiatry is skewed. This does not mean that endogenous biology plays no role, and certainly the biological consequences of obesity are severe and worthy of study. Rather, the problem is a skewed allocation of resources that does not match the scientific evidence about the etiology of obesity on the one hand, or schizophrenia on the other.

Chapter 5

The Efficacy of Antipsychotic Medication

Four decades of data demonstrate consistently and conclusively that antipsychotic medications have only a modest effect on psychotic symptoms. Given that the available medications for psychosis have only modest efficacy, it is important to investigate both the environmental etiology of psychosis and its treatment with psychosocial interventions. Hence my proposal that there is a dissociative subtype of schizophrenia. One purpose of the proposal is to provide a rationale for, data in support of, and a logical structure for serious study of the psychotherapy of psychosis.

I am not saying that psychotherapy is ineffective for nondissociative subtypes of schizophrenia, or that it is effective for all cases of the dissociative subtype. In terms of treatment planning, the purpose of the theory is to identify a subgroup that is *more likely* to respond to psychotherapy.

Just as the genetic model of schizophrenia is refuted by four decades of data, the widespread belief that antipsychotic medications are powerful and effective is merely a belief, one refuted conclusively by the existing data.

In a review, Jibson and Tandon (1998) endorsed the widespread but incorrect belief that neuroleptics are effective medications: "The past few years have witnessed an unprecedented development of new antipsychotic medications. As with their neuroleptic predecessors, these medications are effective in reducing the delusional thinking, hallucinatory experiences, and thought disorganization which are the hallmarks of psychosis" (p. 215).

It is true, based on twin concordance data, that schizophrenia is a genetic disorder—but only to a minor degree. Similarly, it is true that antipsychotic medications are more effective than placebo. This difference is statistically significant. Rather than being robust, however, the difference between antipsychotic drugs and placebo is modest.

They work to a certain extent, but are really effective only in a small subset of patients.

The data from prospective, randomized, placebo-controlled trials have consistently shown that these medications are only marginally superior to placebo, and meta-analyses demonstrating this fact have been available for several decades. For instance, Davis (1980) found that out of sixty-six studies of chlorpromazine, there was no difference between drug and placebo in eleven of the studies. The difference between chlorpromazine and placebo found in fifty-five of the studies was statistically significant but modest in magnitude.

Taiminen et al. (1997) stated that the rate of placebo response in antipsychotic medication trials ranges from 20 to 40 percent. In their own study of forty-five subjects on placebo, they found that 26.7 percent experienced a score reduction of 20 percent or more on the PANSS. The main point of their study was the finding that ratings of response did not differ significantly between fifteen different psychiatrists who viewed videotapes of patient interviews. These findings argued against rater bias as an explanation for the placebo response.

In a review article on quetiapine (Seroquel), Kasper and Muller-Spahn (2000) present a bar graph showing the percentage of subjects responding to various doses of quetiapine in a multicenter, double-blind, randomized, prospective, placebo-controlled study. "Response" was defined as a reduction of 40 percent or greater in scores on the BPRS. The bar graph demonstrates visually that quetiapine is superior to placebo.

However, examination of the y-axis of the bar graph reveals that only 29 percent of subjects responded to the most effective dose of quetiapine, which was 150 milligrams. The bar graph also shows comparison data from a study of olanzapine (Zyprexa). Kasper and Muller-Spahn (2000) point out in their discussion that quetiapine is as effective as olanzapine, which is true statistically. However, they fail to comment on the fact that the percentage of subjects responding to placebo in the olanzapine study was greater than the percentage of subjects responding to the most effective dose of quetiapine.

Meta-analytic data have demonstrated for several decades that the various antipsychotic medications are equally effective if given in equivalent doses. For instance, Davis (1980) reviewed 122 studies published prior to 1980 in which chlorpromazine was compared to one of nineteen other neuroleptics. In none of these 122 studies was the other medication superior to chlorpromazine. The antipsychotic medications differ in side effects, but not in efficacy; therefore efficacy data for any of them are representative of all antipsychotic medications.

Volavka et al. (2002) conducted a randomized controlled trial of clozapine, olanzapine, risperidone, and haloperidol in treatment of chronic schizophrenia and schizoaffective disorder. The reductions in scores on the PANSS over fourteen weeks are shown in Table 5.1. The data demonstrate that all four of these medications have minimal effect on positive symptoms, negative symptoms, and general psychopathology. The only cell in Table 5.1 with a symptom reduction of greater than 10 percent is the response of positive symptoms to olanzapine.

In terms of specificity of action, the antipsychotic medications could just as well be called anti–general psychopathology medications. Their effect on positive and negative symptoms is no more impressive than their effect on general psychopathology.

Positive symptoms of schizophrenia are symptoms that are present but normally would be absent; they include hallucinations, delusions, thought disorder, and agitation. Negative symptoms are the absence of normal attributes; they include reduced drive, social withdrawal, emptiness, and a flat emotional tone. General psychopathology includes anxiety, depression, substance abuse, and other Axis I and II symptoms—on the PANSS, general psychopathology means all psychiatric symptoms other than positive and negative psychotic symptoms.

TABLE 5.1. The efficacy of clozapine (N = 40), olanzapine (N = 39), risperidone (N = 41), and haloperidol (N = 37)

	Reduction in PANSS score		
Medication	Positive symptoms (%)	Negative symptoms (%)	General psychopathology (%)
clozapine	8.9	6.4	5.8
olanzapine	13.2	7.4	9.2
risperidone	9.1	1.7	2.3
haloperidol	6.2	+2.3	2.0

Source: Adapted from Volavka et al., 2002.

Note: PANSS = Positive and Negative Syndrome Scale

Imagine a medication for childhood fever that worked as well as the neuroleptics. If we set normal temperature at 0, then a fever of 102.6°F becomes a temperature of 4. A 20 percent reduction in fever would mean that on the most effective dose of the antipyretic, the child's temperature dropped to 101.8°F. Such an antipyretic would fail in the marketplace. Parents would not buy it.

In a study funded by Eli Lilly and Company, the manufacturers of olanzapine, the senior author, an employee of Eli Lilly, reported on "the beneficial effects of olanzapine in rapidly controlling behavioral agitation" and concluded that "physicians should consider using olanzapine as the first line of therapy in schizophrenia" (Kinon et al., 2002, pp. 19, 20). The conclusion that olanzapine is superior to haloperidol for treatment of agitation in schizophrenia was based on the finding that olanzapine resulted in a reduction of BPRS agitation scores of 25.6 percent compared to 16.4 percent for haloperidol. In fact, the data prove that both drugs are marginally effective and that the effect of the two medications on agitation is indistinguishable clinically.

The Kinon et al. (2002) article is titled, "Effective Resolution with Olanzapine of Acute Presentation of Behavioral Agitation and Positive Psychotic Symptoms in Schizophrenia." It was included as a free insert with the May 2002 issue of the *Canadian Journal of Psychiatry*. It would be more accurately titled, "The Minimal Effect of Olanzapine on Behavioral Agitation and Positive Psychotic Symptoms in Schizophrenia." A 25.6 percent reduction in symptoms cannot represent an "effective resolution" of any clinical problem in medicine or psychiatry.

Arvantis and Miller (1997) conducted a multicenter, randomized, placebo-controlled study of quetiapine versus haloperidol and placebo for the treatment of acute exacerbations of chronic schizophrenia. Their results confirm the modest efficacy of neuroleptics. The most effective dose of quetiapine, 150 milligrams, reduced symptoms on the BPRS by 18.4 percent. Translated into the treatment of fever, this means a reduction in temperature from 102.6°F to 101.9°F. Such a fever still needs treatment. A child with a temperature of 101.9°F would qualify to participate in a study of a new antipyretic. The reductions in BPRS scores at various doses of quetiapine are shown in Table 5.2.

Another way the data are analyzed in drug studies is to perform a *responder analysis*. In the quetiapine study, a responder was defined as anyone whose score dropped by 40 percent or more. Table 5.3 shows that at the most effective dose, 150 milligrams, only 29 percent of subjects were responders. This means that 71 percent of people prescribed quetiapine do not respond.

However, the data are even more unfavorable to quetiapine when one considers the average BPRS score at entry into the study for subjects randomized to 150 milligrams of quetiapine, which was 47.2, as shown in Table 5.2. A subject with an entry score of 47.2 who experiences a drop in BPRS score of 40 percent now has a score of 28.3. Such a subject still scores higher than the BPRS score of 27 required to get into the study. This means that only about 25 percent of sub-

TABLE 5.2. The efficacy of quetiapine—reduction in Brief Psychiatric Rating Scale (BPRS) scores

BPRS score	Placebo (N = 51)	150 mg (N = 48)	300 mg (N = 51)	600 mg (N = 51)
Baseline	45.3	47.2	45.3	43.5
End point	46.7	38.2	36.6	35.9
Change	+1.7	−8.7	−8.6	−7.7
% change	+3.7	−18.4	−19.0	−17.7

Source: Adapted from Arvantis and Miller, 1997.

TABLE 5.3. The efficacy of quetiapine—responder analysis

Reduction in BPRS score (%)	Placebo (N = 51) (%)	150 mg (N = 48) (%)	300 mg (N = 51) (%)	600 mg (N = 51) (%)
>20	16	46	43	45
>40	6	29	25	27
>60	2	13	18	18
>80	0	4	0	6

Source: Adapted from Arvantis and Miller, 1997.

jects given an antipsychotic medication experience a drop in symptoms sufficient to disqualify them for entry into another study.

In order to appreciate the true meaning of these data in the real world, one must consider the inclusion and exclusion criteria for the study. These are invariable, with minor exceptions, throughout the psychopharmacological literature.

The inclusion criteria for the quetiapine study were the requirement that subjects score above 27 on the BPRS, meet DSM-III-R criteria for schizophrenia and score above 4 (moderately ill) on the Clinical Global Impression scale. It is the exclusion criteria that are important. These are the items that exclude subjects from participation.

Exclusion criteria were presence of any other Axis I disorder; seizures; significant medical problems; pregnancy; and use of an injectable neuroleptic within the previous dosing interval (e.g., if the injection is given once a month, within the previous month).

These criteria exclude most schizophrenics in the world and almost all schizophrenics in treatment at psychiatric hospitals. For practical reasons, all schizophrenics who are homeless, in jails, and noncompliant with treatment are also eliminated. The study population, then, for the entire world's literature on psychiatric medications, is hard-to-find, clean, pure cases.

The measure of how hard it is to find such cases of schizophrenia is the number of participating centers required to enroll and complete 361 subjects in the quetiapine study—twenty-six centers. Subjects for drug studies are routinely recruited through radio and newspaper advertisements because it is impossible to find enough of them at treatment centers.

The efficacy of quetiapine, then, is its efficacy in the cleanest, tidiest, easiest-to-treat individuals in the world. I predict that the efficacy of the medication would be even lower with real-world subjects. These include people with depression, substance abuse, anxiety disorders, violent behavior, medical problems, serious head injuries, or attention deficit disorder, as a brief set of examples. A study could be conducted with two groups of subjects: people who meet DSM-IV-TR criteria for schizophrenia and who do not have Axis I comorbidity, and subjects with severe comorbidity including schizophrenia. Both groups would be randomized to active medication and placebo.

I predict that the response of clean, tidy cases to placebo would be equal to or higher than the response of highly comorbid subjects to active medication. If there were specific genetic markers for schizophrenia to incorporate in such a study, I predict that the markers would be found most frequently in the least comorbid subjects, who would also be the best medication responders. They would also have the least psychological trauma.

Table 5.3 shows that 54 percent of subjects who received 150 milligrams of quetiapine experienced less than a 20 percent reduction in BPRS scores. As stated above, only 29 percent experienced a score reduction of 40 percent or more and therefore could be classified as responders. The number whose score dropped by 80 percent or more was only 4 percent, which is no different clinically or statistically from placebo.

Let me clarify how to read Table 5.3. Forty-eight subjects received the 150 milligram dosage of quetiapine. Of the forty-eight subjects, 46 percent experienced score reductions of 20 percent or greater on the BPRS. This 46 percent includes those who experienced score reductions of 60 percent or greater and those who experienced reductions of 80 percent or greater. Similarly, the 13 percent of subjects who experienced score reductions of 60 percent or greater includes those who experienced reductions of 80 percent or greater.

An 80 percent score reduction from an average entry score of 47.2 means an end-point score of 9.4, but this response was attained by only 4 percent of the subjects. Hardly anyone really gets better because of antipsychotic medication, even among the easiest-to-treat, most compliant subjects.

These conclusions are based on the scientific facts. They are irrefutable. They have immediate ethical implications for future studies of the psychotherapy of psychosis. For instance, since the average subject experiences only an 18.4 percent reduction in symptoms due to neuroleptics, withholding medication during a trial of psychotherapy is feasible from an ethical perspective, given that subjects can be dropped out of treatment studies at any time.

If medications were withheld from all subjects in a study of psychotherapy for schizophrenia, the small percentage of subjects who are robust responders to medication would be denied effective treatment. However, this group would be counterbalanced by the robust responders to psychotherapy who would not receive effective psychotherapy under standard clinical conditions. In any case, subjects are already randomized to placebo in drug trials; therefore the decision to withhold treatment from robust responders has already been made by ethics committees throughout the world.

Extreme ethical objections about withholding medications in studies of the psychotherapy of schizophrenia would not be consistent with the scientific facts. The medications are not powerful and effective, except in a small subset of subjects who cannot be identified in advance by current approaches to schizophrenia.

One purpose of the theory of a dissociative subtype of schizophrenia is to identify a subgroup more likely to respond to psychotherapy. The inverse purpose is to separate out nondissociative subjects who may be more likely to respond to medication. If the criteria for dissociative schizophrenia can in fact make this distinction with good sensitivity and specificity, then the ethical burden of withholding medication would become higher in nondissociative schizophrenia than in the dissociative subtype. In other words, the theory may better protect a subgroup of subjects who are medication responders than does current practice.

The ethics of placebo-controlled trials in schizophrenia were reviewed by Carpenter, Appelbaum, and Levine (2003). These authors concluded that it is ethical and acceptable to randomize subjects to placebo in drug studies of schizophrenia. Thus studies comparing active medication alone, psychotherapy alone, a combination of medication and psychotherapy, and a combination of psychotherapy plus placebo medication would be ethical.

Carpenter, Appelbaum, and Levine (2003) make four points concerning use of placebo in drug studies for schizophrenia:

1. The medications affect primarily positive symptoms, but long-term outcome is primarily affected by negative symptoms and cognitive deficits. Therefore, withholding medication during a study should not affect long-term outcome.
2. Other beneficial treatments need not be withheld in the placebo condition.
3. Subjects who are poor responders to medication are not deprived of benefit.

4. Nonresponders can be dropped from the study at any time or active medication can be added to their treatment on a nonblind basis. The addition of active nonstudy medication is itself a variable of interest and can be analyzed statistically.

My argument that it is ethically feasible to assign subjects with schizophrenia to psychotherapy alone is consistent with the views and analysis of Carpenter, Appelbaum, and Levine (2003). They are recognized authorities on schizophrenia and their article was published in the *American Journal of Psychiatry.*

Critical analyses of psychiatry and psychopharmacology usually focus on the cost side of the cost-benefit analysis (Wiseman, 1995; Whitaker, 2001). Such authors emphasize the toxicities, side effects, drug-drug interactions, and other costs of neuroleptics, antidepressants, psychostimulants, and anxiolytics. Analysis of the benefit side of the equation, however, demonstrates that only modest costs are required to yield a negative cost-benefit ratio (Ross and Read, 2004).

The world's psychopharmacological literature on antidepressants is similar to that for antipsychotics. For instance, in a review of seventy-five methodologically rigorous trials of antidepressants published in the English literature from 1981 to 2000, Walsh et al. (2002) found that overall, 30.0 percent of depressed subjects respond to placebo while 50.1 percent respond to antidepressants. In these studies, "response" was defined as a 50 percent reduction in depression scores. Similar to the findings for neuroleptics, the difference between antidepressants and placebo is statistically significant but modest in magnitude, and half of subjects do not respond to medication.

In the same issue of the *Journal of the American Medical Association,* Davidson (2002) reported a study of sertraline versus St. John's wort and placebo in the treatment of depression. There was no difference between St. John's wort and placebo, or between sertraline and placebo. This is the same pattern that we see in the neuroleptic literature—many rigorous studies that find no difference between drug and placebo. The difference that emerges from meta-analyses is modest.

Lecrubier et al. (2002) compared St. John's wort (N = 186) to placebo (N = 189) and found the active medication to be more effective. This was true statistically at $p < .04$. However, the average drop in Hamilton Rating Scale for Depression (HAM-D) scores was 9.9 for

St. John's wort and 8.1 for placebo, a difference that has no clinical meaning.

Summarizing the antidepressant literature, Tranter et al. (2002, p. 243) stated that "a third of patients achieve complete remission, a third do not respond and a third show partial remission." Kennedy et al. (2002, p. 270), writing in the same issue of the *Journal of Psychiatry and Neuroscience,* stated that "only 25 percent-35 percent of patients experience full remission" on antidepressants.

Cascalenda, Perr, and Looper (2002) performed a meta-analysis of six studies in which antidepressant medication (N = 261), psychotherapy (N = 352), and a control or placebo treatment (N = 270) were compared. They found rates of full remission of 46.4 percent for medication, 46.3 percent for psychotherapy, and 24.4 percent for placebo. Full remission was defined as scores below 7 on the HAM-D in two studies, below 6 in three studies, and below 5 in one study. Thus, although rates of full remission were higher than the 25 to 35 percent cited by Kennedy et al. (2002), the overall pattern was typical: for moderately depressed outpatients, psychotherapy alone and medication alone are equal; both are superior to placebo; and the gap between treatment and placebo is not very large.

An example of an antidepressant study in a special population is the report of Glassman et al. (2002). They studied 369 patients recruited from forty outpatient cardiology centers and psychiatry clinics in seven countries. All subjects had either a recent myocardial infarction (74 percent) or unstable angina (26 percent). They were randomized to sertraline versus placebo.

Both groups had average HAM-D scores of 19.6 at entry. After two weeks of single-blind placebo run-in, subjects received either drug or placebo on a double-blind basis for twenty-four weeks. At the end of the study, the average HAM-D score for subjects receiving sertraline was 11.2, while for placebo it was 12.0 ($p = .14$). Sertraline reduced HAM-D scores by only 0.8 points more than did placebo.

On a post hoc basis, the authors divided the subjects into three groups: those with two or more prior major depressive episodes and initial HAM-D scores above 18 (a severe group); those with any number of prior depressive episodes irrespective of baseline HAM-D scores (an intermediate group); and those with no prior history of depression (a mild group).

The severe group had reductions in HAM-D scores of −12.3 compared to −8.9 for placebo ($p = .01$), while the intermediate group had reductions of −9.8 for sertraline and −7.6 for placebo ($p = .009$). These were the positive results that proved that sertraline is effective for treatment of depression in the population under study.

However, only 90 subjects out of 369 (24.4 percent) belonged to the severe group, while 75.6 percent belonged to the intermediate or mild groups. Among three-quarters of the subjects, the average reduction in HAM-D scores due to sertraline was less than two points greater than the reduction due to placebo.

Glassman et al. (2002) concluded that for " 'more severe' patients, sertraline was found to be robustly superior to placebo." They elsewhere described sertraline as "effective" and concluded that acute coronary syndrome "should be identified and treated because it is a serious illness" (pp. 707, 708).

A commentary on the study (Carney and Jaffe, 2002, p. 751) concluded, "We hope that the results of this important study will encourage physicians to recognize and appropriately treat depression in patients with heart disease."

The study was funded by Pfizer, the manufacturer of sertraline, and the final author, Dr. Harrison, is an employee of Pfizer who participated in the design, analysis, and reporting of the data. A major conclusion of the study was that there was no difference between sertraline and placebo on all cardiovascular outcome measures; therefore, sertraline was found to be "safe and effective" for people with recent heart attacks or unstable angina.

Glassman et al., 2002 used the lack of difference between drug and placebo on cardiovascular outcome measures to prove that the medication is safe. In this safety analysis, they used all subjects. When they followed the same procedure to establish efficacy (using all patients in the study), they again found no difference between drug and placebo. The type of analysis that established safety also demonstrated a lack of efficacy.

This is the reason that the authors undertook a subanalysis of the more severely depressed subgroup—they needed to find a statistically significant antidepressant effect in a subgroup that would support their claim of efficacy. Otherwise, there would be no point in prescribing the medication. The authors reported on the greater efficacy of sertraline in the severe group but did not say whether there was a difference in safety between drug and placebo in the severe group.

To be consistent, the authors should also have reported on the safety of the medication in the severe group. Perhaps this analysis was unfavorable and was suppressed. This study resulted in endorsements of sertraline as effective and robustly superior to placebo that are not consistent with the data. Overall, no difference was found between sertraline and placebo in the Glassman et al. (2002) study. In the small subgroup for whom a statistically significant difference occurred between sertraline and placebo, the medication reduced HAM-D scores by less than two points more than did placebo. It is impossible that "robustly superior" is a scientifically accurate assessment of the data in Glassman et al. (2002).

No evidence shows that antidepressant medications affect the rates of attempted and completed suicide, at either the general population level or the individual case level. There are no double-blind trials of antidepressants in which attempted and completed suicide were tracked as treatment outcome measures, and in which an antidepressant was found to differ from placebo (Oquendo et al., 2002). In fact, current suicidal ideation is an exclusion criterion in Phase III antidepressant trials. Therefore, the world's double-blind placebo-controlled data on antidepressants do not directly address the question of the effect of antidepressant medications on attempted and completed suicide.

In a meta-analysis of the Federal Food and Drug Administration database on antidepressant clinical trials, Khan, Warner, and Brown (2000) found that active antidepressants do not differ from placebo in their effects on rates of attempted and completed suicide.

The data from the antidepressant literature resemble the findings for antipsychotic medications. The research is funded by drug companies. The difference between drug and placebo is modest, and claims of efficacy are far out of proportion to the data.

It is a logical error to infer from the efficacy of medications that the illness being treated is therefore an endogenous, biomedical disease. For instance, aspirin can be effective for reducing fever when the fever is caused by a biologically normal response to a virus. However, if we accept, for the sake of argument, that the efficacy of neuroleptics is a measure of the degree to which psychosis is an endogenous biomedical disease, the data are clear: psychosis is an endogenous biomedical disease only to a modest degree.

A simple calculation reduces the gap between medication and placebo even further. Consider the antidepressants. Overall, 50 percent of subjects respond to antidepressants and 30 percent respond to placebo. This means that, of the subjects who respond to medication, 30 percent would have done just as well if they had been randomized to placebo; 70 percent of the responders to medication actually required the chemical effect of the medication to get that response.

This means that only 35 percent ($0.5 \times 0.7 = 0.35$) of all subjects given antidepressants respond in a manner attributable to the pharmacological effect of the medication. This is barely more than the 30 percent who respond to placebo. The world's data on antidepressants and antipsychotics therefore support the conclusion that depression and psychosis are induced by the psychosocial environment and the meaning of human experience, as much as they support the conclusion that psychiatric problems are induced by internal biological variables.

The world literature on psychopharmacology is consistent with the postulates underlying the dissociative subtype of schizophrenia. Antipsychotic medications are only marginally effective and there is a pressing need for research on psychosocial treatment strategies (Bustillo et al., 2001). Of course, there are many possible explanations for the modest efficacy of antipsychotic medications; it is possible in principle, for instance, that all cases of schizophrenia have endogenous biological causes, but existing medications do not target the core pathophysiology.

The lack of efficacy of antipsychotic medications proves nothing about the etiology of schizophrenia. My point is this: since the medications don't work very well, common sense suggests a greater investment in trials of psychotherapy; also, to repeat, although lack of medication efficacy proves nothing about etiology, it is consistent with the theory that in a substantial subset of cases, schizophrenia is not an endogenous biomedical illness. If this is correct, excluding individuals with dissociative schizophrenia from medication trials, or analyzing them separately, might increase the gap between medication and placebo in the remaining subjects.

My theory has an inverse benefit: if it identifies an environmentally induced subgroup that is more responsive to psychotherapy, it may also define, by exclusion of dissociative subjects, a predominantly endogenous disease subgroup with a better response to medication and more easily identifiable endogenous pathophysiology, including genetic defects. I am not opposed to the endogenous biological etiology of schizophrenia on principle; the existing data do not support that model for schizophrenia overall, but I predict that it does apply to a subgroup, once subjects with dissociative schizophrenia are excluded.

If we are to practice evidence-based medicine, as I think we should, we need to acknowledge the conclusive evidence: the existing antipsychotic medications don't work very well. This is true of antidepressants, anxiolytics, and other classes of medication as well. The difference between antipsychotic medications and placebo is statistically significant in many studies, but modest. The majority of subjects in the literature do not respond to antipsychotic medication.

Chapter 6

Psychosis and Trauma

John Read
Colin A. Ross

The majority of people who meet DSM-IV-TR criteria for schizophrenia have suffered major trauma at some point in their lives (Goodman et al., 1999; Lysaker et al., 2001). Therefore the majority of such individuals could benefit from being offered the full range of psychological and psychosocial treatment modalities for psychological trauma (Follette, Ruzek, and Abueg, 1998; van der Kolk, McFarlane, and Weisath, 1996), even if the trauma played no direct etiological role in the psychosis.

The experience of psychosis and the accompanying hospitalizations, takedowns, involuntary commitments, enforced intramuscular injections, loss of contact with the outside world, legal problems, and other negative consequences are themselves a major trauma (Lundy, 1992; Meyer et al., 1999; Shaw, McFarlane, and Bookless, 1997; Shaw et al., 2002). Such trauma could perpetuate the psychosis or make it worse, even if it was not the initial cause of it (Sautter et al., 1999).

High rates of trauma are also observed in schizotypal personality disorder, which is often considered to be a variant of schizophrenia. Yen et al. (2002) reported a 56.0 percent lifetime rate of PTSD. Of these eighty-six subjects, 29.1 percent reported childhood sexual abuse, 40.0 percent childhood physical assault, 39.5 percent involvement in a serious accident, and 47.7 percent witnessing a serious injury or killing; altogether 84.9 percent reported some type of trauma history.

In this chapter I review the evidence for an etiological link between psychological trauma and psychosis. The possibility of a traumatic etiology for the dissociative subtype of schizophrenia is supported by a large body of data.

CHILDHOOD TRAUMA AND GENERAL PSYCHOPATHOLOGY

Adult disorders for which child abuse and neglect have been shown to be significant risk factors include depression, anxiety disorders, PTSD, eating disorders, suicidality, substance abuse, sexual dysfunction, personality disorders, and dissociative disorders (Beitchman et al., 1992; Boney-McCoy and Finkelhor, 1995; Brodsky et al., 2001; de Graaf et al., 2002; Kendler et al., 2000; Levitan et al., 1998; Macmillan et al., 2001). Childhood abuse is also strongly linked to many of the leading causes of death in adults, including ischemic heart disease, cancer, stroke, chronic bronchitis or emphysema, and diabetes (Felitti et al., 1998).

The more severe the abuse, the greater the probability of a psychiatric disorder in adulthood (Fleming et al., 1999; Mullen et al., 1993). Although it is clear that the effects of childhood trauma are not uniquely linked to psychotic symptoms, the literature reviewed next indicates that the relationship of childhood trauma to schizophrenia may be at least as strong, and perhaps stronger, than the relationships of childhood trauma to other less severe disorders in adulthood.

Compared to other psychiatric patients, those who suffered childhood physical abuse (CPA) or childhood sexual abuse (CSA) are more likely to attempt suicide, have earlier first admissions and longer and more frequent hospitalizations, spend more time in seclusion, receive more medication, and exhibit higher global symptom severity (Beck and van der Kolk, 1987; Beitchman et al., 1992; Briere et al., 1997; Bryer et al., 1987; Goff et al., 1991; Pettigrew and Burcham, 1997; Read, 1998; Sansonnet-Hayden et al., 1987). One study found that CSA was a more powerful predictor of adult suicidality than a current diagnosis of depression (Read, Agar, et al., in press).

THE BASE RATE OF CHILD ABUSE AMONG PSYCHIATRIC INPATIENTS

In thirteen studies of "seriously mentally ill" women, the percentage that experienced either CSA or CPA ranged from 45 to 92 percent

(Goodman et al., 1997). Another review of fifteen studies totaling 817 female psychiatric inpatients calculated that 64 percent reported either CPA or CSA, with 50 percent reporting CSA and 44 percent reporting CPA (Read, 1997). A study of girls in a child and adolescent psychiatric inpatient unit found that 73 percent had suffered either CSA or CPA (Ito et al., 1993). Read (1997) concluded that women in psychiatric hospitals are at least twice as likely as other women to have been abused as children. This may be a conservative estimate because general population studies, which often involve multiple screenings and extended interviews, tend to produce higher and more accurate rates (Jacobson, 1989), and because psychiatric inpatients tend to underreport abuse (Dill et al., 1991; Read, 1997; Read and Argyle, 2000).

Male inpatients report rates of CPA similar to those of their female counterparts (Rose, Peabody, and Stratigeas, 1991; Jacobson and Richardson, 1987). Male inpatient CSA rates range from 22 to 39 percent, with a female-to-male ratio ranging from 2.3:1 to 1.3:1 (Jacobson and Herald, 1990; Rose, Peabody, and Stratigeas, 1991; Sansonnet-Hayden et al., 1987; Wurr and Partridge, 1996). Male inpatient CSA rates are at least double the rates of CSA in the general male population in England (Palmer et al., 1994) and the United States (Jacobson and Herald, 1990).

Prevalence rates in a mixed-gender sample of child and adolescent inpatients (21 percent of whom were diagnosed with a psychotic disorder) were: CSA, 37 percent; CPA, 44 percent; emotional abuse, 52 percent; emotional neglect, 31 percent; and physical neglect, 61 percent (Lipschitz et al., 1999). The CSA had a mean age of onset of 8 years and a mean duration of 2.1 years. The majority of the CSA was intrafamilial and involved penetration or oral sex. The CPA had a mean age of onset of 4.4 years, lasted an average 6.4 years, and involved physical injury in the majority of cases.

Craine et al. (1988) studied rates of childhood sexual abuse among 105 female patients at a state hospital; 43 of the women had a primary diagnosis of schizophrenia, 23 an affective disorder, and 7 other psychoses. Of the 105 women, 51 percent had been abused sexually, and 66 percent met criteria for PTSD, although none had received that diagnosis clinically. Of those who reported sexual abuse, only 20 percent believed they had received adequate treatment for the sexual abuse.

When the subjects were divided into those reporting sexual abuse (N = 54) and those not reporting sexual abuse (N = 51), the abused women had significantly higher rates of self-mutilation, severe reactions to pelvic exams, compulsive sexual behavior, sadomasochistic sexual fantasies, sexual identity conflicts, chemical dependency, homosexuality, gagging responses, preoccupation with sexual matters, and a number of other symptoms.

A large body of data demonstrates conclusively that psychiatric inpatients, many of whom are psychotic, report high rates of psychological trauma, including childhood physical and sexual abuse.

CHILDHOOD TRAUMA AND PSYCHOSIS

Among the recent advances identified by the British Psychological Society (Kinderman, Cooke, and Bentall, 2000) is the finding that "many people who have psychotic experiences have experienced abuse or trauma at some point in their lives" (p. 28). A growing body of research demonstrates this finding in relation to schizophrenia and child abuse.

Rosenberg et al. (2001) reviewed relevant studies on psychological trauma in individuals with severe mental illness published from 1970 to 2000. They concluded, "People with severe mental illness have a markedly elevated risk of exposure to trauma" (p. 1455). Specifically, between 34 and 53 percent report childhood physical or sexual abuse, while between 43 and 81 percent report having experienced some type of victimization.

Four studies of female inpatients or outpatients with predominantly psychotic diagnoses found incest prevalences from 22 percent to 46 percent, with a total of 112 out of 397 (28 percent) reporting incest (Beck and van der Kolk, 1987; Cole, 1988; Muenzenmaier et al., 1993; Rose, Peabody, and Stratigeas, 1991).

CSA and CPA are significantly related to research measures of psychosis in general and schizophrenia in particular. "Psychoticism," as measured on the Symptom Checklist 90-Revised (SCL-90-R), was found, in female inpatients, to correlate more strongly than any of the other clinical scales with abuse history (Bryer et al., 1987). "Psychoticism" discriminates more powerfully ($p < .001$) than any of the other SCL-90-R scales between men who had and had not been abused as children (Swett, Surrey, and Cohen, 1990). The psychoticism scale also correlates more strongly with the number of perpetrators of CPA and CSA than any of the other SCL-90-R scales (Ellason and Ross, 1997b).

Both the SCL-90-R Psychoticism scale and Minnesota Multiphasic Personality Inventory (MMPI) Schizophrenia scales differentiate incest victims and nonabused women (Lundberg-Love et al., 1992; Scott and Stone, 1986). Adults who suffered CPA score significantly higher than others on both the Paranoia and Schizophrenia scales of the MMPI-2 (Cairns, 1998). Chronically mentally ill women who have been abused score higher than those who have not been abused on the Beliefs and Feelings scale, measuring psychotic symptoms (Muenzenmaier et al., 1993).

CSA is also related, in the general population, to the unusual experiences component (including perceptual aberrations) of schizotypy (Startup, 1999). Perceptual Aberration scale scores, which are predictive of clinical psychoses, are ten times more common in young adults who were maltreated as children than those who were not maltreated (Berenbaum, 1999).

Individuals who have received a diagnosis of schizophrenia as adults are significantly more likely than the general population to have run away from home (Malmberg, Lewis, and Allebeck, 1998), attended child guidance centers (Ambelas, 1992), and been placed in children's homes (Cannon et al., 2001). In a thirty-year study of 524 child guidance clinic attendees, 35 percent of those who developed schizophrenia as adults had been removed from their homes because of neglect, which was twice as many as any other diagnostic group (Robins, 1966). Among women inpatients diagnosed with schizophrenia in one study, 60 percent had suffered CSA (Friedman and Harrison, 1984). Among chronically hospitalized psychotic women in another study, 46 percent had suffered incest (Beck and van der Kolk, 1987).

In a mixed-gender sample of adults diagnosed with schizophrenia, 83 percent had suffered CSA, CPA, or emotional neglect (Honig et al., 1998). A chart review found that 48 percent of women inpatients diagnosed with schizophrenia (but only 6 percent of the men) had suffered definite or probable CSA, and that 52 percent of the women and 28 percent of the men had suffered definite "parental violence" (Heads, Taylor, and Leese, 1997). Of 5,362 children in another study, those whose mothers had poor parenting skills when they were four years old were significantly more likely to develop schizophrenia as adults (Jones et al., 1994).

Parental hostility precedes, and is predictive of, schizophrenia (Rodnick et al., 1984). In families in which both parents expressed high levels of criticism toward their child, 91 percent of disturbed but nonpsychotic adolescents were diagnosed (within five years) as having schizophrenia or a related disorder; whereas in families in which both parents were rated low on criticism, only 10 percent of similarly disturbed but nonpsychotic adolescents were diagnosed as psychotic (Norton, 1982).

A community survey in Winnipeg, Canada (N = 502) found that 45.7 percent of those with three or more Schneiderian symptoms of schizophrenia had experienced CPA or CSA, compared to 8.1 percent of those with none (Ross and Joshi, 1992). The CPA, CSA, and Schneiderian symptoms inquired about in this study were operationalized in the structured interview used in the study, the Dissociative Disorders Interview Schedule (DDIS). The DDIS has sufficient reliability and validity to be included in the American Psychiatric Association's *Handbook of Psychiatric Measures* (Pincus et al., 2000), and psychometric data and the text of the interview schedule are available in Ross (1997). The DDIS is also available at <www. rossinst.com>. Thus, the definitions of abuse and psychotic symptoms in this study were well operationalized.

The sample of subjects was derived from a stratified cluster sample of the general population that closely matched census data for the city of Winnipeg. The sampling procedure and demographics of the subjects are described in Ross and Joshi (1992) and Ross, Joshi, and Currie (1990). This study and its conclusions, then, are based on a valid general population sample, a valid and reliable structured interview, and operationalized definitions of abuse and psychotic symptoms.

In the 502 subjects, the number of Schneiderian symptoms correlated at $p < .00001$ with sexual and/or physical abuse ($r = .32$), the number of perpetrators of physical abuse reported ($r = .21$), the number of perpetrators of sexual abuse reported ($r = .25$), and the number of types of sexual abuse reported ($r = .19$). In a regression analysis with the number of Schneiderian symptoms as the criterion variable, physical and/or sexual abuse had a beta weight of 0.51 as a predictor variable (F ratio $= 23.337$, $p < .0001$). This study provides evidence that childhood physical and sexual abuse are significant risk factors for later psychotic symptoms.

Inpatients who suffered CSA or CPA are significantly more likely than other inpatients to experience voices commenting, paranoid ideation, thought insertion, ideas of reference, visual hallucinations, or reading others' minds (Ross, Anderson, and Clark, 1994). An outpatient study found that hallucinations, across all sensory modalities, are significantly more common in patients who suffered either CSA or CPA than those who did not (Read, 2001). In a Dutch study, 65 percent of individuals with schizophrenia related the initial onset of hearing voices to traumatic events such as witnessing people being shot in a war, the suicide of a close family member, and CSA and CPA. Furthermore, "the disability incurred by hearing voices is associated with (the reactivation of) previous trauma and abuse" (Honig et al., 1998, p. 646).

Hallucinations have been found to be particularly common among incest survivors (Ensink, 1992). Ellenson (1985) identified, in forty women, a "post incest syndrome," including hallucinations, which he reported as "exclusively associated with a history of childhood incest" (p. 526). This was replicated in ten other incest cases (Heins, Gray, and Tennant, 1990). Read and Argyle (1999) found that all female incest survivors in their inpatient study experienced hallucinations and that incest survivors were significantly more likely to do so than those subjected to extrafamilial CSA.

One might ask whether these symptoms were hallucinations or flashbacks. It is a question of definition and mind-set (see Table 11.1). When these symptoms occur in a population regarded as suffering from an endogenous biomedical psychosis, they are classified as hallucinations. When the same symptoms occur in a population regarded as suffering from trauma-induced disorders, they are classified as flashbacks. Just as psychosis and dissociation are not discrete categories, so too hallucinations and flashbacks overlap a great deal and are often the same thing.

Both parental absence and institutionalization in childhood are related to schizophrenic symptoms later in life, with a particularly strong relationship, for boys, to thought disorder, hallucinations, delusions, and hebephrenic traits (Walker et al., 1981).

Not only do abused psychiatric patients experience schizophrenic symptoms more often than nonabused patients, they do so at a younger age (Goff et al., 1991). Among children admitted to a psychiatric hospital, 77 percent of those who had been sexually abused were diagnosed as psychotic, compared to 10 percent of those who had not been abused (Livingston, 1987). Adolescent inpatients who have experienced CSA are more likely to hallucinate than those who have not (Sansonnet-Hayden et al., 1987). Famularo, Kinscherff, and Fenton (1992) found that hallucinations were significantly more likely in a group of severely maltreated five- to ten-year-olds than in a control group, in keeping with an earlier study (Ensink, 1992), which found that "the content of the reported visual and/or auditory hallucinations or illusions tended to be strongly reminiscent of concrete details of episodes of traumatic victimization" (p. 126). Read and Argyle (1999) found the content of 54 percent of schizophrenic symptoms in adults to be similarly related to child abuse. Examples included command hallucinations to self-harm in the voice of the perpetrator.

Read, Agar, et al. (in press) reported data from a sample of 200 clients at community mental health centers; sexual or physical abuse was described in the medical records of 92 of the clients. The most common primary diagnoses among the 200 subjects included depression (N = 85), schizophrenia (N = 28), substance abuse (N =20), and bipolar mood disorder (N = 15). Several types of auditory hallucination were more common among the abused clients ($p < .001$), including voices commenting and command hallucinations.

The relationship between child abuse and psychiatric sequelae in adulthood remains after controlling for potentially mediating variables such as socioeconomic status, marital violence, parental substance abuse and psychiatric history, and other childhood traumas (Boney-McCoy and Finkelhor, 1995; Downs and Miller, 1998; Fleming et al., 1999; Kendler et al., 2000; Pettigrew and Burcham, 1997). After controlling for factors related to disruption and disadvantage in childhood, women whose CSA involved intercourse were twelve times more likely than nonabused females to have had psychiatric admissions (Mullen et al., 1993).

Among women at a psychiatric emergency room, 53 percent of those who had suffered CSA had "nonmanic psychotic disorders (e.g., schizophrenia, psychosis NOS)" compared to 25 percent of those who were not victims of CSA; corresponding findings for CPA were 49 and 33 percent (Briere et al., 1997, p. 96.) After controlling for "the potential effects of demographic variables, most of which also predict victimization and/or psychiatric outcome," CSA was related to nonmanic psychotic disorders ($p < .001$) and depression ($p < .035$) but not to manic or anxiety disorders (Briere et al., 1997, p. 99).

Research into the pathways linking childhood trauma to psychotic symptoms later in life needs to be a higher priority within psychiatry. We already know of remarkable similarities between dysfunction and damage found in the brains of traumatized children and in the brains of many adults with schizophrenia (Read, Perry, et al., 2001). Another promising area for research into the relationship between trauma and psychosis is cognitive attributions (Bentall and Kaney, 1996; Barker-Collo, 2001).

The high rate of psychological trauma in individuals with psychosis is demonstrated by a large literature. The data on monozygotic twin concordance for schizophrenia lead to the conclusion that the environment plays a significant role in the causation of schizophrenia, beyond being a mere trigger. Psychological trauma, as defined in the literature on PTSD, is a candidate form of toxic environmental input contributing to the etiology of psychosis, and as such warrants clinical and research attention.

FAILURE OF MOST RESEARCH ON SCHIZOPHRENIA TO CONSIDER PSYCHOLOGICAL TRAUMA

Schizophrenia is widely considered to be an endogenous biomedical disorder (Chua and Murray, 1996; McGuffin et al., 1994; Walker and Diforio, 1997). However, the evidence supporting this proposition is far from conclusive (Bentall, 1990; Boyle, 1990; Jay, 2001; Karon, 1999; Rose, 1991; Ross and Pam, 1995; Turkheimer, 2001), just as it is for other disorders (Goldberg, 2001).

The widely accepted diathesis-stress model of schizophrenia (Norman and Mallar, 1993a,b; Walker and Diforio, 1997) is characterized as a biopsychosocial approach, implying an integration of data from various paradigms. However, the assumption that the diathesis is a diagnostically specific genetic predisposition has curtailed the study of trauma, neglect, and loss by positioning all psychosocial factors exclusively in the stress component of the diathesis-stress model.

Proponents of the diathesis-stress model argue that individuals with schizophrenia are not exposed to disproportionate amounts of stress, but merely overrespond to stress. It is this oversensitivity, or "vulnerability," that is supposedly inherited. Thus, while the diathesis-stress model allows that hostility from family members can cause relapse by activating an "underlying autonomic hyperarousal" (Tarrier and Turpin, 1992) or "neurocognitive vulnerability" (Rosenfarb et al., 2000), the causes of the vulnerability are rarely sought in the interpersonal domain (Norman and Malla, 1993a).

The preconception that the diathesis in the diathesis-stress model is genetic led Norman and Malla (1993a), along with many other reviewers, to include only those studies measuring stressors a few weeks prior to the outbreak of symptoms. Describing this period as "prodromal" allows even these events to be seen as relevant only insomuch as they exacerbate premorbid behavioural dysfunction or, at most, hasten the onset of the initial clinical episode (Walker and Diforio, 1997). McGuffin et al. (1994) have even argued, using hypothetical nontransmissable changes in gene structure or expression, that the environment has no causal role at all, even as a precipitant of symptoms.

The extent to which the widely held diathesis-stress model is, as its name and its proponents suggest, an integration of the biological, the psychological, and the social can be examined by comparing the quantity of research into various possible etiological factors (measured by entries in PsycINFO). Although the three categories of genetics, biochemistry, and neuropsychology combined have, as a proportion of all schizophrenia research, remained quite stable (7.2 percent in the 1960s, 8.0 percent in the 1990s), the proportion of studies investigating stress peaked at 1.2 percent in the 1980s and declined to 0.8 percent in the 1990s.

Schizophrenia research dealing with child rearing or parent-child relationships never attained more than a 1.6 percent share of the total research, in the 1960s, and declined to 0.2 percent in the 1990s. In the last four decades of the twentieth century, for every study on the relationship between child abuse or neglect and schizophrenia, there were thirty on the biochemistry of schizophrenia and forty-six on its genetics. Since 1960, schizophrenia research has accounted for 10.9 percent of the 11,777 research studies appearing in PsycINFO under the heading "Genetics." The figures for psychosocial factors include stress, 0.9 percent of 34,504 studies; socioeconomic status, 0.8 percent of 13,362 studies; and child abuse, 0.1 percent of 10,294 studies.

Research into childhood schizophrenia (McKenna, Gordon, and Rapaport, 1994; Spencer and Campbell, 1994) and reviews of the research (Stabenau and Pollin, 1993; Volkmar, 1996) ignore any stressors beyond birth trauma and viral infection. PsycINFO records that not one of the 19,099 studies conducted before 2001 on child abuse, sexual abuse, physical abuse, emotional abuse, child neglect, or family violence was related to childhood schizophrenia.

Tsuang and Faraone (2002); Tsuang, Stone, and Faraone (2002); and Faraone et al. (2002) reviewed the literature on possible strategies to prevent schizophrenia. Childhood trauma is not mentioned in any of these three articles. Faraone et al. (2002) devoted one paragraph to psychosocial factors and concluded that "communication deviance" in parents who adopt children out of schizophrenic pedigrees can increase the likelihood of thought disorder in the adopted child. Child abuse and neglect were not mentioned.

The only high-risk populations Faraone et al. (2002) identified for possible early intervention were children from schizophrenia pedigrees, children with prodromal signs of schizophrenia, and children who were exposed to pregnancy and birth complications. Other than parental communication deviance, the psychosocial environment plays no role in risk analysis or possible early intervention, according to these authors.

Studies that retrospectively examine the childhoods of adults diagnosed as schizophrenic search for and find evidence of "significant childhood behavioural dysfunction" (Neumann et al., 1995), but the findings are explained in terms of the "constitutional vulnerability" underlying schizophrenia.

A recent study (Cannon et al., 2001) does investigate quality of relationships with parents in childhood but groups this variable under "symptoms," with the implication that any disturbance in the relationship is a result of the illness rather than a possible cause. The fact that the children who were diagnosed with schizophrenia as adults were 2.7 times more likely than children who were not mentally ill as adults to have been in an institution or children's home (a finding absent for those with affective psychosis as adults) seems to raise no questions for these researchers about the role of the environment in causation of schizophrenia.

Malaspina et al. (2001) demonstrated that after controlling for gender and age, traumatic brain injury (TBI) is significantly related ($p < .008$) to a diagnosis of schizophrenia but not to bipolar disorder or major depression. These authors found that 17 percent of adults diagnosed with schizophrenia had suffered TBI. Despite having access to the details of the TBIs, including the patients' age at the time and the nature of the injury, no mention is made by these authors of whether the injuries were accidental or purposefully inflicted. The only explanations considered are whether TBIs "cause a phenocopy of the genetic form of schizophrenia" or "lower the threshold for expressing schizophrenia in those with genetic vulnerability" (p. 441).

One in eight children in the United States between the ages of ten and sixteen has experienced aggravated assault (physical assault involving either use of a weapon or injury), excluding violence within the family (Boney-McCoy and Finkelhor, 1995). A possible relationship between any TBIs resulting from these assaults and subsequent schizophrenia is covered, however, by the statement, "Early illness features of schizophrenia such as agitation or psychosis might increase exposure to traumatic brain injury. If that is true then the head injury does not cause the schizophrenia" (Malaspina et al., 2001, p. 441).

The diathesis-stress model, in its current form, with its insistence that the diathesis to psychosis is predominantly or exclusively genetic, has thus far failed to produce a balanced integration of the research literature on trauma, including TBI (accidental or intentional), neglect, loss, deprivation, and sexual abuse. In its currently prevailing form, the diathesis-stress model is not a truly integrated biopsychosocial model, because within it the fundamental cause of psychosis is biological and unidirectional; the abnormal genome causes a "chemical imbalance," which causes symptoms. The environment is at most a trigger.

Curiously, the diathesis-stress model requires an assumption that many of its adherents would likely reject: for the "stress" to be relevant, even as a trigger, it must be true that toxic input from the psychosocial environment can activate the gene or genes for schizophrenia. If this is true, then one must consider seriously the possibility that input from the psychosocial environment can turn the genes off and deactivate the phenotype.

When people who have received a diagnosis of schizophrenia are asked about the etiology of their symptoms, they respond differently than psychiatrists. Holzinger et al. (2002) analyzed transcripts of interviews with seventy-seven people who were being treated for schizophrenia with clozapine. Of the seventy-seven patients, 48.4 percent mentioned psychosocial stress factors as causes of their illness; 31.2 percent mentioned conditions during childhood or in the parental home; 24.3 percent mentioned personality factors, most often personal sensitivity; 16.7 percent mentioned heredity; 15.4 percent mentioned an illness of the central nervous system; and 14.1 percent mentioned alcohol and drug consumption.

These may be reasonably accurate estimates of the relative contributions of the different etiological factors operating in schizophrenia. I propose that the role of the psychosocial environment is greater among people treated with clozapine than among people receiving other antipsychotic medications, because people receiving clozapine more frequently meet criteria for the dissociative subtype of the disorder.

This prediction is based on a simple piece of logic. I stated in Box 2.1 that reduced response to antipsychotic medication is a characteristic of dissociative schizophrenia. Patients must fail to respond to adequate trials of at least two conventional antipsychotics before they can begin a trial of clozapine. They are by definition poor responders to conventional antipsychotics; therefore they may tend to have the dissociative subtype of schizophrenia.

The postulates underlying the dissociative subtype of schizophrenia are supported by a large body of data and are consistent with the views of people who know schizophrenia from the inside, that is, patients in treatment for schizophrenia. The data are derived from many different methodologies, measures, and research agendas. They are international in scope and published in reputable journals. Additional research findings supporting the relationship between trauma and psychosis are reviewed in subsequent chapters.

PART III:
DISSOCIATION AND DISSOCIATIVE IDENTITY DISORDER

Chapter 7

Definition and Scientific Status
of Dissociation

This chapter itemizes and corrects a number of logical and scholarly errors about dissociation and DID. The errors are discussed under separate headings. For the dissociative subtype of schizophrenia to be a valid diagnostic category, dissociation must be an operationalized concept with a solid scientific foundation.

ERRORS OF LOGIC AND SCHOLARSHIP
CONCERNING DISSOCIATION

Using Dissociation and Repression As Synonyms

Equating dissociation with repression is a scholarly and logical error that must be corrected in order for the dissociative subtype of schizophrenia to be valid. This error is found in writings by McHugh (1997), Ofshe and Watters (1994), Piper (1997), and Spanos (1996). It is true, as these authors argue, that there is no scientific evidence for the intrapsychic defense mechanism of repression as defined by Freud. If repression is synonymous with dissociation, it follows that there is no scientific evidence for dissociation. It then follows that there is no scientific foundation for the dissociative disorders or the dissociative subtype of schizophrenia.

To refute the idea that dissociation equals repression, one must define both terms, which have multiple meanings. Repression has three meanings in the professional literature:

1. *Primal repression,* an unconscious ego defense against unacceptable id impulses and wishes (Freud, 1963). This meaning of repression has nothing to do with trauma, outside events, or memory.

2. *Repression proper,* an unconscious defense mechanism used by the ego to push unacceptable thoughts, feelings, and memories down into the id, or unconscious (Freud, 1963).

3. *A synonym for suppression,* which is consciously putting thoughts or problems on the back burner (Beardslee and Vaillant, 1997).

Dissociation has four meanings of dissociation in the professional literature. The common thread in these four meanings is the core meaning of the word: dissociation is the opposite of association. It is a disconnection between variables. When the executive self is disconnected from the reality of the body, we call that *depersonalization.* When the executive self is disconnected from a memory that normally would be retrievable, we call that *amnesia.* The fundamental idea is a dissociation or disconnection between variables that would normally be linked, interacting, or connected with each other. The four meanings of dissociation follow.

1. The operational definition of dissociation can be found in measures such as the Dissociative Experiences Scale (DES) (Bernstein and Putnam, 1986), the DDIS (Ross, 1997), the Multidimensional Inventory of Dissociation (MID) (Dell, 2002), and the Structured Clinical Interview for DSM-IV Dissociative Disorders (SCID-D) (Steinberg, 1995). The operational meaning of dissociation is based on the same rules and procedures that are applied to measurement of anxiety, depression, or psychosis and is supported by over 250 data-based peer-reviewed publications using the DES, and numerous publications using the DES, DDIS, and SCID-D (Dell, 2002; Ross, 1997). The DES and the pathological dissociation it measures are unifactorial constructs (Bernstein et al., 2001; Dell, 2002). The operationalized meaning of dissociation is the one used to define the dissociative subtype of schizophrenia: dissociation is the items in measures of dissociation.

2. The general systems meaning of dissociations or disconnections between variables, are understood and measured mathematically in all areas of science, including general medicine (Ploghaus et al., 1999). In this meaning, dissociation is the opposite of association—it is a disconnection or lack of interaction between variables. This general meaning of dissociation is common to all four meanings of the word.

3. Dissociation is a technical term in cognitive psychology (Cohen and Eichenbaum, 1993). Dissociations between procedural and declarative memory have been studied in cognitive psychology experi-

ments for decades. Subjects have included normal college students, brain-damaged humans, and experimental animals. Dissociation within long-term memory is one of the most rigorously demonstrated phenomena in cognitive psychology. This is the literature relevant to the scientific status of dissociation. The authors cited previously ignore it or are unaware of it. It is a proven scientific fact that accurate memory of real events can be present in procedural memory and can affect verbal and behavioral output in a measurable fashion, in the complete absence of conscious memory of that information. Contrary to the cited authors' claims, this phenomenon does not depend on special mechanisms or assumptions such as "robust repression" or "repression theory." It is a proven aspect of the psychological function of the normal human mind.

4. Dissociation is a defense mechanism postulated to be used to cope with traumatic events (Putnam, 1989, 1997).

It is possible that the fourth meaning of dissociation could be a synonym for the second meaning of repression; however, it is not. As defined by Hilgard (1977), dissociation involves vertical splitting. Traumatic information is never pushed down into the unconscious mind. It is pushed across a vertical barrier into another compartment of the ego or conscious mind. It is never "repressed." Repression occurs when material is pushed downward across a horizontal split into the unconscious mind, where it is not available for conscious recall. Hilgard's use of the term *repression* corresponds to Freud's *repression proper.*

Initially, in his book *Studies on Hysteria* (Breuer and Freud, 1986 [1895]; Ross, 1997), Freud subscribed to a trauma-dissociation theory. Women patients came to him with childhood sexual abuse memories and a wide variety of symptoms. He viewed the dissociated components of the abuse memories as the cause or drivers of the symptoms. He assumed the memories to be real. They were held in split-off compartments of the ego. This was the same theory espoused by Pierre Janet (1965 [1907], 1977 [1901]) in the same time period. Freud called his theory the seduction theory. Treatment involved reintegrating the dissociated information and feelings.

In the late 1890s, as reflected in his letter to Wilhelm Fleiss on September 21, 1897, Freud repudiated the seduction theory (Masson, 1985). He decided that the sexual abuse memories were false. In order to explain why his women patients were presenting to him with false memories of childhood sexual abuse and myriad symptoms, he developed repression theory. It is when memories are judged to be false that repression theory applies.

Freud broke with Janet. Dissociation theory and repression theory are separate, different things. That is why the word *repression* does not appear in the DSM-IV-TR and why there is no section called Repression Disorders. It is why the DSM-IV-TR has a diagnosis of dissociative amnesia but not one of repressed memories or repressive amnesia. The difference between repression and dissociation is the reason why Freudian psychoanalysts do not diagnose DID, according to Spanos (1996).

Dissociative amnesia is based on conclusive findings in cognitive psychology. It assumes the scientifically proven memory processes of the normal human mind, not any special or unusual theory. A diagnosis of dissociative amnesia is an observation. The phenomenon of dissociative amnesia, that is, a dissociation between procedural and declarative memory, is a fact of normal psychology. The diagnosis is based also on the judgment that this particular instance of dissociative amnesia is too extensive to be explained by ordinary forgetting. One explanation is ruled out by the DSM-IV-TR criteria, but no other one is required, since the diagnosis is phenomenological, not mechanistic.

Recovery of "Repressed Memory"

Several authors claim that there is no scientific evidence for the accurate recovery of repressed memory (Ofshe and Watters, 1994; Piper, 1997; Pope et al., 1999; Spanos, 1996). Based on the erroneous idea that repression equals dissociation, these authors then use the absence of scientific evidence for recovery of repressed memories as evidence against the validity of the dissociative disorders and their treatment.

This argument is erroneous because the idea that repression equals dissociation is incorrect, because the validity of a disorder does not depend on the validity of its treatment, and because abundant scientific evidence shows that the normal human mind can recover accurate memories for which it was previously amnesic. Remembering something that has been unavailable but on the tip of your tongue is a common example.

A large body of scientific literature in cognitive psychology demonstrates the reality of cued retrieval (Cohen and Eichenbaum, 1993). Subjects are given memorization tasks and later are asked to recall as much of the task information as possible. They have imperfect recall in this situation, which is called spontaneous recall, unassisted recall, or free recall. Subjects are then given clues about information they have not remembered in the free recall situation. They now report more accurate information for which, in clinical terms, they previously had amnesia. This is called cued retrieval.

The inability to recall information prior to cueing is proof of the reality of dissociative amnesia. An amnesia, or inability to recall, is reversed by a simple verbal stimulus. The reversal requires a prior dissociation between procedural and declarative memory, accurate storage of the information in procedural memory, and successful transfer of the information to declarative memory in response to the cue.

Calling these operations an example of the reversal of dissociative amnesia does not require an assumption about the retrieval mechanism. Cued retrieval is a proven fact of normal human psychological function, not a theory or belief. Recovery of accurate memories is an inevitable outcome of any psychotherapy involving presentation of retrieval cues by the therapist or repeated recall effort by the patient (Erdelyi, 1996).

There is abundant experimental information about the conditions internal and external to the subject during a recall task that both augment and inhibit accurate retrieval (Erdelyi, 1996). Abundant data also exist on the original stimulus variables that affect cued retrieval, including duration of stimulus presentation, type of stimulus, clarity of the stimulus, emotional valence or meaning of the stimulus, and so on.

Recovery of memory in therapy is simply an example of cued retrieval. The accuracy and error rate of the recovered, cued material is an empirical question. Abundant evidence shows that the simple repeated effort to recall results in the retrieval of more information than was previously available to conscious memory.

When the effect of simple effort to recall is controlled for experimentally, hypnosis adds nothing to the subject's recall performance. Hypnosis in and of itself does not increase the quantity of either accurate or inaccurate memories recovered, independently of simple repeated recall effort (Erdelyi, 1996). The controversy about recovered memories and their accuracy has minimal if any relevance to the scientific status of dissociation.

Relevance of Repression Theory to the Scientific Status of DID or Dissociative Schizophrenia, or Standards of Care for Treatment

Studies by Herman and Schatzow (1987); Williams (1994); Briere and Conte (1993); Feldman-Summers and Pope (1994); Loftus, Polonsky, and Fullilove (1994); and other studies reviewed by Brown, Scheflin, and Hammond (1998) and Brown, Scheflin, and Whitfield (1999) deal with the phenomenon of recovered memory but do not address dissociation as such. Conclusive relevant science concerning dissociation is contained in the experimental cognitive psychology literature (Cohen and Eichenbaum, 1993; Ross, 1999).

For instance, *repetition priming* is an example of the operation of dissociation in the normal human mind, as is *task interference*. A typical repetition priming experiment involves *homophonic word pairs,* which sound the same but are spelled differently and have different meanings, such as *bear/bare* and *reed/read*. Normal subjects are presented with lists of homophonic word pairs, which they memorize. Later, in a free recall situation, they are asked to write down as many word pairs as they can remember, but most cannot remember *reed/read*. In clinical terminology, they have amnesia for the experience of memorizing *reed/read*.

The subjects are then asked to write down the answer to a question that invokes one word in the word pair, for example, "What is the name of a tall, thin, tubular aquatic plant that grows in marshes?" Students who have been exposed to the *reed/read* word pair spell the answer incorrectly as *read* more often than control subjects who did not have the *reed/read* word pair in their lists.

Repetition priming demonstrates the proposition that accurately held information about real events can be stored in the unconscious mind and affect verbal and behavioral output in a scientifically measurable fashion, in the complete absence of conscious memory for that information. The experimental cognitive psychology literature on the reality of dissociation is voluminous and conclusive. The scientific status of dissociation is confirmed by clinical psychiatry and the DSM-IV-TR, but is not dependent on it.

Dissociative amnesia in response to trauma does not require any special cognitive operations peculiar to traumatic memory, nor any neuropsychological mechanisms from outside normal human psychology. Nontraumatic, accurate memory of real events is routinely held in procedural memory, where it is unavailable to declarative memory without specific cueing. The name for this phenomenon in long-term memory is *dissociation*.

Arguments about the theory of repression are relevant to the diagnosis and treatment of DID and dissociative schizophrenia only if those disorders depend on repression theory, but they don't. There are Freudian, repression-based theories for almost every diagnosis in the DSM-IV-TR. Freudian psychoanalysts have tried to treat just about every disorder in the DSM-IV-TR using methods based on repression theory. The reliability and validity of the dissociative subtype of schizophrenia and the efficacy of its treatment are empirical questions that do not require Freud. This is true for dissociative schizophrenia as it is for all disorders on Axis I and II.

As formulated, the Freudian defense mechanism of repression is not scientifically testable. I am not saying that Freudian theory is wrong, nor am I saying that psychoanalytical therapies are ineffective. My point is that the scientific status of dissociation is solid and independent of repression or other Freudian theories.

Dissociation and Hypnosis

Many authors equate dissociation with hypnotizability (McHugh, 1997; Ofshe and Watters, 1994; Piper, 1997; Spanos, 1996). They further equate being highly dissociative with being highly suggestible since, for them, dissociative equals hypnotizable equals suggestible. Being highly suggestible is then said to be a vulnerability to iatrogenic DID. There are several errors in these logical steps.

First, scores on the DES and standard measures of hypnotizability correlate at about $r = 0.14$ in nonclinical populations (Whalen and Nash, 1996). Hypnotizability and dissociation are separate constructs. The existing science clearly refutes the idea that dissociation equals hypnotizability.

Many authors claim that highly dissociative people are necessarily highly suggestible. This claim, advanced by Ofshe and Watters (1994) and Piper (1997), is not supported by any scientific evidence. The

only empirical study on the question (Leavitt, 1997) shows a correlation between DES and suggestibility scores of $r = 0.17$.

I elaborate on the etiology of DID and the controversy about its
iatrogenesis in a later chapter. Skeptics about DID who consider most
or all cases to be iatrogenic, and those who consider it to be a naturally occurring trauma disorder, are in agreement on one fundamental
point: all parties consider the disorder, to be a reaction to the environment. Disagreement is limited to age at onset and disputes about
which environment activates the disorder, the family of origin or the
therapy provided to the adult patient.

High hypnotizability is an element of the operationalized definition of the dissociative subtype of schizophrenia, along with numerous other features. However, no scientific evidence supports the hypothesis that the dissociative subtype of schizophrenia is an artifact of
hypnotizability or suggestibility. Such misconceptions have been applied to DID; I analyze them here in an attempt to prevent their application to dissociative schizophrenia.

DIAGNOSIS OF DISSOCIATIVE IDENTITY DISORDER

Errors of logic and scholarship about the diagnosis and treatment
of DID could be repeated in critiques of the dissociative subtype of
schizophrenia; therefore, arguments against those errors are presented here. The errors of logic could also be applied to forms of
chronic, complex dissociation subsumed under the DSM-IV-TR category of dissociative disorder not otherwise specified (DDNOS), but
they have been applied only to DID by skeptics. Therefore I limit my
analysis to DID, although it encompasses partial forms of DID,
which are accounted for within the category of DDNOS. My concern
is to refute errors of logic before they are applied to the dissociative
subtype of schizophrenia.

The Claim That DID Cannot Be Diagnosed Reliably

Piper (1997, p. 28) claims that the DSM-IV criteria for DID are
vague and asks, "That is, how do MPD theorists determine that the
disorder is *not* present?"

There are abundant data on methods for determining that DID is
not present using clinical interviews, the DES, the DDIS, the MID

(Dell, 2002), or the SCID-D (Ross, 1997). Nine studies in five countries finding an average prevalence of undiagnosed DID of 4 percent among general adult psychiatric inpatients are not reviewed by Piper—they show that DID is not present in 96 percent of cases, according to the DDIS, SCID-D, and clinicians (Ross, 1997). The methods for determining that DID is not present are well documented, replicated, and reliable.

How would depression or any other DSM-IV disorder be shown to be absent? The scientific rules for establishing the specificity, sensitivity, reliability, and validity of psychiatric diagnoses are well defined, and apply to both DID and the dissociative subtype of schizophrenia. Piper (1997) claims that the DSM-IV definition of DID is vague but never examines the actual reliability data. One could make the same critique of any DSM-IV criteria set, for instance substance abuse, that requires "clinically significant impairment or distress" (American Psychiatric Association, 1994, p. 182). Who is to say what is "clinically significant"?

Depression (APA, 1994, p. 327) requires "depressed mood most of the day, nearly every day." How are "most" and "nearly" defined, and how depressed does "depressed" have to be?

Reliability is demonstrated by scientific studies of interrater reliability. These have defined rules and methodology that apply to all diagnoses. Virtually all criteria sets in the DSM-IV-TR could be made to look vague and subjective using analysis of the semantics of their criteria sets. Piper's (1997) criticisms of the DSM-IV criteria for DID are semantic, not scientific or methodological. It is possible that a vaguely worded criterion set could result in poor reliability. This can be determined only if the necessary reliability research has been done. Otherwise, the claim that vague wording has caused poor reliability is simply an untested hypothesis.

Piper (1997) has not subjected his hypothesis to scientific tests, nor has he specified how this could be done. He does not use the existing data to test it, and has never conducted any research himself. The claim that the DSM-IV criteria for DID generate false positives is a hypothesis worthy of study, but not a fact. The published reliability data on DID show that it has reliability as good or better than the average for Axis I (Ross, 1997).

There are numerous such errors of scholarship in Piper (1997). For instance, the SCID-D, developed by Marlene Steinberg, is not discussed and Steinberg is not referenced. The SCID-D was developed in the mid-1980s. Data on it were first published in 1990 by Steinberg, Rounsaville, and Cicchetti (1990). A book on it was published by the American Psychiatric Press in 1995 (Steinberg, 1995), and the SCID-D research was funded by the National Institutes of Mental Health. The SCID-D cannot be ignored in any scientific discussion of the reliability of DID.

DID and the other dissociative disorders are valid and reliable according to the scientific and evidence-based criteria applied to psychiatric disorders in general. That is why they are included in the DSM-IV-TR and in the American Psychiatric Association's *Handbook of Psychiatric Measures* (Pincus et al., 2000). To appear in that text, measures had to be scrutinized and approved by reviewers and committees. None of the editors of the text has ever published work on dissociation or the dissociative disorders, and none has any demonstrable bias in favor of their inclusion in the text.

The Dissociative Taxon and Pathological Dissociation

Dissociation is understood clinically according to both continuum and discrete category models, which are not mutually exclusive. Looked at one way, the data support the conclusion that dissociative experiences in the general population occur on a continuum from normal through mild to severely pathological dissociation (Ross and Joshi, 1992). However, when taxometric analysis is applied to the data (Waller and Ross, 1997), a discrete category of pathological dissociation emerges.

Piper (1997) and other authors who reject the validity of DID (Ofshe and Watters, 1994; McHugh, 1997; Merskey, 1995; Simpson, 1995; Spanos, 1996) must account for the procedure of taxometric analysis and its application to the DES (Waller, Putnam, and Carlson, 1996; Waller and Ross, 1997). Taxometric analysis of DES scores divides general population and clinical samples into two discrete categories with little or no overlap: normal versus pathological dissociation. The taxometric data establish that pathological and normal dissociation can be differentiated with high levels of scientific reliability, and thereby provide a fundamental foundation for the reliability and validity of the dissociative subtype of schizophrenia. The subtype could not be valid if the construct of dissociation was not valid.

I am not saying that the reliability and validity of the DES-Taxon (DES-T) provide evidence that dissociative schizophrenia is a valid category. I am saying that demonstrated validity of the category of pathological dissociation is a necessary foundation or precondition for the validity of dissociative schizophrenia.

Examples of normal dissociation include staring off into space and missing part of a conversation. Such experiences are nearly universal, occur occasionally, and cause no serious impairment or distress. They could become pathological if their frequency increased, however, for instance, if one spent 80 percent of the day in a trance state. Other experiences, in contrast, are inherently pathological and are rare in the general population. Most people never experience them. Examples include not recognizing oneself in the mirror, or not recognizing close friends or family members.

DID and pathological dissociation are psychiatric categories that can be differentiated from normal with high levels of sensitivity and specificity. I discuss the continuum versus discrete state models of pathological dissociation further in the next chapter.

Failure to Understand the Rules of the DSM System

Several authors state that DID is not a valid psychiatric disorder, based on their rejection of the childhood trauma model of DID (McHugh, 1997; Merskey, 1995; Ofshe and Watters, 1994; Piper, 1997; Simpson, 1995; Spanos, 1996). This opinion is based in part on the previously noted errors of logic about repression. In addition, the authors have failed to grasp the rules of the DSM system (DSM-III, DSM-III-R, DSM-IV, and DSM-IV-TR have the same rules). The DSM-IV-TR diagnostic criteria sets are phenomenological. They are not based on theories of causality, which are irrelevant to the reliability and validity of DSM-IV-TR disorders, as is the efficacy of treatment. This is true throughout medicine. For instance, cancer of the pancreas is a valid diagnosis, even though no one knows its cause and there is no treatment.

Reliability is demonstrated through studies and data. The rules for these studies, which are standard for all disorders, have been applied to the dissociative disorders using the DES, DDIS, SCID-D, and MID (Dell, 2002; Ross, 1997). Pope and Hudson (1992), authors skeptical of the validity of the dissociative disorders, nevertheless state that the DDIS has established reliability.

Disagreement about etiological theories of DID is irrelevant to discussion of the reliability of the disorder. The DSM-IV-TR does not differentiate iatrogenic from trauma-induced DID. Patients judged to have iatrogenic DID still meet DSM-IV-TR criteria and receive the diagnosis by DSM-IV-TR rules. These are the rules for making psychiatric diagnoses of the relevant scientific community, namely the American Psychiatric Association.

Inclusion of a disorder in the DSM-IV-TR does not, by itself, prove the scientific validity of the disorder. However, inclusion represents the authoritative judgment of the relevant scientific community. It is therefore within the standard of care to make that diagnosis. Inclusion of a disorder provides strong evidence in favor of the inverse proposition: for a disorder to appear in the DSM-IV-TR, there can be no conclusive scientific proof available in the literature that it lacks acceptable reliability and validity.

Environmental etiology is inherent in my model of the dissociative subtype of schizophrenia. However, it is perfectly possible, in principle, that a predominantly genetic form of schizophrenia could meet symptom criteria for the dissociative subtype. Even if a history of reported severe, chronic trauma was incorporated as a diagnostic criterion for dissociative schizophrenia in future editions of the DSM, clinicians making the diagnosis would not have to assume that the trauma caused the disorder.

Consistent with general DSM rules, I have made a report of chronic trauma a phenomenological criterion for dissociative schizophrenia (see Chapter 14). No assumption about the etiological role of the trauma is required under this approach. Clinicians can reject a trauma etiology, accept it, or regard it as provisional, and in all three instances can endorse the validity of the dissociative subtype at the same level and in the same way as they accept all other DSM categories.

For the reasons described, I favor including a history of childhood trauma as one item in a polythetic criterion set for dissociative schizophrenia, rather than as a required item. The criterion set for dissociative schizophrenia should not be constructed the same way as for PTSD. PTSD absolutely requires the presence of trauma in Criterion A to make a diagnosis. I propose making the trauma criterion for dissociative schizophrenia one item in a polythetic criterion set in order to allow for a nontrauma pathway to the subtype. There is no reason, in principle, why dissociative schizophrenia cannot be caused by endogenous disease in some cases.

Lack of Evidence in Support of the Theory of Iatrogenic Dissociative Identity Disorder

Spanos (1996) performed experiments in which normal college students acted as though they had DID when he asked them to do so. He regarded this as evidence in favor of the iatrogenic theory of DID. Spanos himself differentiates between *simulation* and *role enactment*. Simulation is conscious and deliberate and corresponds to clinical factitious DID. Role enactment is not deliberate, is truly believed in by the person doing the enactment, and is unconscious. Role enactment corresponds to clinical iatrogenic DID.

Spanos (1996) says that iatrogenic DID is based on role enactment. The therapist gives the cues and suggestions necessary for the iatrogenic patient to enact the role. Spanos states that iatrogenic DID is not based on simulation.

Spanos's college students simulated DID. They never believed they really had it—otherwise Spanos would have created iatrogenic DID on purpose, which would have been unethical, harmful, and grounds for a lawsuit. The college student data on simulation of DID are irrelevant to the claim that DID is a role enactment in patients who develop it through iatrogenic causation.

GENERAL ERRORS OF LOGIC AND SCHOLARSHIP

Skeptical opinions about the validity of DID are fueled by a series of general errors of logic and scholarship. I review them here because these classes of erroneous argument could be applied to the dissociative subtype of schizophrenia.

Using an Observation to Prove a Hypothesis

The logical error of using an observation to prove a hypothesis is pervasive in the writings of authors who reject the validity of DID. For instance, it is an agreed-upon fact that more cases of DID are diagnosed inside North America than outside, by far. Similarly, more cases were diagnosed in the 1980s and 1990s than previously, by far (Merskey, 1995; Piper, 1997; Simpson, 1995; Spanos, 1996).

In science, a researcher makes an observation, then forms a hypothesis, then conducts an experiment or some form of research to test the hypothesis. The two competing hypotheses in this instance are (1) DID is iatrogenic versus (2) DID is naturally occurring. If DID is iatrogenic, the epidemic is limited primarily to North America. If DID is regarded as naturally occurring, the prediction is that DID is equally common outside North America but is underdiagnosed.

The authors just cited use the observation that DID is diagnosed less often outside North America as proof of their hypothesis that it is iatrogenic. They thereby violate the basic rules of scientific method. In fact, the observation is neutral and equally compatible with both hypotheses. The only way to tell which hypothesis is correct is with science, that is, by conducting research or experiments that provide data for or against the two competing hypotheses. The authors cited provide no data of their own and ignore or distort the existing data (Akyuz et al., 1999) or simply dismiss it without analysis.

The question of the prevalence of DID in other countries, clinical populations, and the general population is epidemiological. The scientific rules and procedures for answering such questions are well established.

Confusing Phenomenon with Mechanism

When dissociative amnesia and repression are equated, logical categories are being confused. Dissociative amnesia is not a theory. It is an observation. The doctor observes the patient reporting inability to remember important personal information, usually of a traumatic or stressful nature, that is too extensive to be explained by ordinary forgetfulness. Thousands of patients made this claim to thousands of psychiatrists throughout the twentieth century, for numerous kinds of trauma including verified events (Loewenstein, 1993).

The DSM-IV-TR criteria do not assume any cause or mechanism. When the phenomenon of dissociative amnesia is observed, the defense mechanism of repression is only one possible cause.

Contradictions Between Skeptical Authors' Views of Freud

A number of authors who reject the validity of dissociation and DID cite one another as authorities. However, they contradict one another in their views of Freud. Piper (1997), McHugh (1997), and Ofshe and Watters (1994) attack Freud and his theories. They characterize recovered memory therapy as based on unscientific Freudian repression theory. They also endorse Spanos's college student experiments as evidence against the validity of DID and regard Spanos as authoritative in his analysis of DID.

Spanos (1996), however, states that adherence to Freudian theory protects the therapist against creation of iatrogenic DID. He states that trauma dissociation theory was rejected by Freud and argues that repression theory steers the therapist away from personification of ego states or a belief in dissociation within the ego. This contradiction reveals yet another error of scholarship among professionals skeptical of DID.

This chapter has reviewed and analyzed some of the most common errors of logic and scholarship concerning dissociation, DID, repression, and alleged false memories. Additional analysis of these and related errors is contained in other sources (Barton, 1994a,b; Braude, 1995; Brown, 2002; Brown, Scheflin, and Hammond, 1998; Brown, Scheflin, and Whitfield, 1999; Cheit, 2002; Dallam, 2002a,b; Dickstein, Riba, and Oldham, 1997; Gleaves, 1996; Kluft, 1998; Martinez-Taboas, 1995; Pezdek and Banks, 1996; Pope, 1996, 1997; Putnam, 1995; Ross, 1997; Tice et al., 2002; Whitfield, 2002; Whitfield, Silberg, and Fink, 2002; Whittenburg et al., 2002). Together with this chapter, these sources provide a substantial and scholarly counterargument to critiques of dissociation, the dissociative disorders, and psychotherapy for them.

Chapter 8

Dissociation and Trauma

In this chapter I review evidence that pathological dissociation is often a response to psychological trauma. In my 1989 text (Ross, 1989), I proposed that dissociation can be divided into four domains: normal biological, abnormal biological, normal psychological, and abnormal psychological. Similar schemes have since been proposed by Cardena (1994), Hilgard (1994), and Kihlstrom (1994), among others. These four domains can exist in pure form but usually overlap and co-occur. In this chapter, as in the rest of the book, I focus on abnormal psychological dissociation.

Symptoms of the dissociative subtype of schizophrenia are likely both biological and psychological in origin. Biological and psychological are not discrete categories because endogenous brain disease can cause psychological symptoms and psychological trauma can cause damage to hippocampal neurons (Bremner, 2002; Bremner, Vermetten, et al., 1998; Heim and Nemeroff, 1999; Markowitsch et al., 1998; Teucher-Noodt, 2000) and to other biological systems including neurotransmitters and the hypothalamic-pituitary-adrenal axis (Newport, Stowe, and Nemeroff, 2002; Nijenhuis, van der Hart, and Steele, 2002).

A number of levels and types of evidence support the hypothesis that pathological dissociation is a response to psychological trauma. Before reviewing them, I discuss the problem of whether a continuum or a discrete state model applies to pathological dissociation.

A CONTINUUM OF DISSOCIATION VERSUS DISCRETE PATHOLOGICAL STATES

Some dissociative experiences are in and of themselves normal, and must occur at a high frequency to cause distress or interfere with function. Staring off into space and missing part of a conversation is a normal dissociative experience covered by the DES and is probably a mixed biological-psychological phenomenon. Although this experience is common and normal, it would be pathological if it occurred 80 percent of the time.

People with chronic, complex dissociative disorders report that they experience the normal DES items at high frequencies. Most people report experiencing them 0 to 10 percent of the time. Thus, people with DID have normal dissociative experiences but to an abnormal degree.

Other dissociative experiences are inherently abnormal and are reported by only a small segment of the general population. These include the eight items that make up the DES-T (Waller, Putnam, and Carlson, 1996; Waller and Ross, 1997). The DES-T items are shown in Table 8.1.

Very few people report experiencing these eight DES-T items. Scores on these items are divided into two dichotomous categories: 0 percent of the time versus 5 percent of the time or more. People with DID often endorse frequencies of 30 percent or more for these items.

The procedure of taxometric analysis provides a statistically derived DES-T profile. Almost all subjects score at or near zero on the DES-T and are said to be nontaxon members. A small number of subjects in the general population, about 3 percent (Waller and Ross,

TABLE 8.1. Pathological dissociative experiences from the Dissociative Experiences Scale-Taxon (DES-T)

DES-T item	DES-T item no.
Finding oneself in a place but unaware how one got there	3
Find new things among belongings but do not remember buying them	5
See oneself as if looking at another person	7
Do not recognize friends or family members	8
Feeling that other people, objects, and the world are not real	12
Feeling that one's body is not one's own	13
Feeling as though one were two different people	22
Hearing voices inside one's head	27

1997), have taxon scores near 1.0 and are taxon members. There are very few ambiguous or intermediate cases; therefore taxometric analysis divides subjects into two discrete categories with high reliability: normal versus pathological dissociation.

Similar logic and analysis could be applied to measures of anxiety, depression, psychosis, substance abuse, pathological eating, gambling, and all other DSM categories. To date, only the DES has been subjected to such analysis, but the same principles could be applied to all forms of psychopathology.

The experience of hearing voices talking out loud inside one's head is included in the DES-T. However, it is also reported by a small number of individuals with no demonstrable psychopathology (Honig et al., 1998). It is the only DES-T item that I would exclude from the dissociative taxon on clinical grounds for a small number of individuals. Otherwise, the eight DES-T items are clearly pathological at both clinical and statistical levels.

Bernstein et al. (2001) provided a series of statistical arguments in favor of the conclusion that the DES measures a single dimension. They state that, "the DES is a unidimensional instrument within the context of a factor analytic model" (p. 12). Thus, both the continuum and discrete pathological state models apply to the DES. When the procedure of taxometric analysis is applied, pathological dissociation can be differentiated from normal with high reliability. However, when factor analytic methods are used, dissociation is a continuum and the DES measures a single, unified dimension.

This is similar to the logic of the wave-particle duality in physics. Under some experimental conditions, light functions as a particle, while under other conditions it functions as a wave. Three things are simultaneously true: everyone has normal dissociative experiences on occasion; people with dissociative disorders have the same experiences more frequently; and there are inherently pathological experiences that define a discrete dissociative taxon. The relationship between trauma and dissociation applies to both forms of dissociation: normal experiences occurring to an abnormal degree, and intrinsically pathological experiences.

The existence of a modern psychometric literature on dissociation makes it possible to investigate and establish the scientific validity of the dissociative subtype of schizophrenia. This was not possible before 1985 because that literature did not exist then. Part of the purpose of this book is to bring students of schizophrenia up to date on the dissociation literature.

THE TRAUMA-DISSOCIATION MODEL

The Volume of Scholarly Work on Trauma and Dissociation

The relationship between dissociation and trauma has been the subject of sixteen edited volumes in the last two decades (Braun, 1986; Bremner and Marmar, 1998; Cohen, Berzoff, and Elin, 1995; Klein and Doane, 1994; Kluft, 1985; Kluft and Fine, 1993; Krippner and Powers, 1997; Lynn and Rhue, 1994; Michelson and Ray, 1996; Quen, 1986; Sanchez-Planell and Diez-Quevedo, 2000; Silberg, 1996; Singer, 1990; Spiegel, 1993, 1994; Spira, 1996). During this period, a large number of single- or multiple-author books on the subject have also been published (see Ross, 1997). In addition to sixteen single- or multiple-author books listed in my 1997 text, there have been volumes by Bremner (2002), Chu (1998), Nijenhuis (1999), Putnam (1997), and Rivera (1996). In addition, in my 1997 text I list five special editions of professional journals dealing with dissociation. All of this literature is academic and scholarly in nature.

During this period, two professional journals have specialized in dissociation, *Dissociation* (1988-1997) and its successor, the *Journal of Trauma and Dissociation* (2000-present). The 2004 meeting of the International Society for the Study of Dissociation was its twenty-first consecutive annual meeting. These books, journals, and meetings are evidence of two decades of serious scholarly study of trauma and dissociation.

Although the existence of this scholarly literature does not in and of itself provide proof of a link between trauma and dissociation, it demonstrates that the linkage has been taken seriously by a large group of scholars. The literature provides conclusive evidence that the trauma-dissociation link has face validity for a community of scholars.

The International Character of the Literature on Trauma and Dissociation

If the literature on the link between trauma and dissociation were limited to North America, its validity and generalizability would be in doubt. In the past decade, however, the literature has become international in scope. The greatest empirical contributions have come from Turkey (Akyuz et al., 1999; Sar, Yargic, and Tutkun, 1996; Tutkun et al., 1998), Belgium (Vanderlinden, 1993), and the Netherlands (Boon and Draijer, 1993; Friedl and Draijer, 2000; Nijenhuis, 1999).

The DES and the two structured interviews for dissociative disorders have been translated into numerous languages. I have spoken on trauma and dissociation at conferences and workshops in Spain, Belgium, the Netherlands, Norway, Germany, China, and Australia. This provides a measure of the level of international interest in the subject.

Epidemiological studies of dissociation in clinical and nonclinical populations have been conducted in Canada (Horen, Leichner, and Lawson, 1995; Ross, 1991; Ross, Anderson, et al., 1991; Ross, Ryan, et al., 1991), the United States (Latz, Kramer, and Hughes, 1995; Murphy, 1994; Rifkin et al., 1998; Ross, Duffy, and Ellason, 2002; Saxe et al., 1993), France (Darves-Bornoz, Degiovanni, and Gaillard, 1995; El-Hage et al., 2002), Norway (Knudsen et al., 1995), Turkey (Akyuz et al., 1999; Sar et al., 1996; Tutkun et al., 1998), China (Ross, Keyes, and Xiao, 2002), Switzerland (Modestin et al., 1996), Japan (Berger et al., 1994), the Netherlands (Friedl and Draijer, 2000), Germany (Gast et al., 2001), and Belgium (Vanderlinden, 1993). In addition, structured interview profiles of large groups of individuals with dissociative disorders have been collected in Australia (Middleton and Butler, 1998) and systematic clinical profiles in Puerto Rico (Martinez-Taboas, 1989).

Cross-cultural studies of dissociation have also been conducted in Hawaii (Haugen and Castillo, 1999), Germany (Huber, 1995), and Bali (Suryani and Jensen, 1993), and cross-cultural aspects of dissociation have been discussed in Spiegel (1994), Sanchez-Planell and Diez-Quevedo (2000), and Krippner and Powers (1997). These sources are only a sampling of the total literature and are illustrative but not exhaustive.

There is consistent replicated evidence that dissociative disorders, including dissociative identity disorder, can be diagnosed in a wide range of cultures and languages. The hypothesis that pathological dissociation is diagnosed only in North America or is a culturally limited North American phenomenon (Merskey, 1995; Simpson, 1995), is refuted by a substantial empirical literature. No studies have been conducted outside North America using valid and reliable measures of dissociation that failed to find pathological dissociation and dissociative disorders.

Coons et al. (1991) identified twenty-three countries in which multiple personality disorder has been diagnosed. These countries, plus China, are listed in Box 8.1. In addition, members of the International Society for the Study of Dissociation (ISSD) include professionals from Argentina, Denmark, Finland, Guam, the Phillipines, South Africa, and South Korea. It is unlikely that these individuals would join the ISSD if they had not seen pathological dissociation in their practices.

Two of the hallmarks of pathological dissociation, both contained in the DES-T, are switches of executive control and amnesia. These are also the hallmarks of possession states, which are universal and have been described in numerous sources for more than 2,000 years. There is no doubt that human beings have exhibited the core symptoms of pathological dissociation in countless cultures for thousands of years. I assume that a wide range of possession, trance, ecstatic,

---

BOX 8.1. Countries in which dissociative identity disorder has been diagnosed

Australia	England	Japan
Belgium	France	Mexico
Brazil	Germany	New Zealand
Bulgaria	Guatemala	Puerto Rico
Canada	Holland	South America
China	India	Spain
Columbia	Israel	Switzerland
Czechoslovakia	Italy	United States

and dissociative states throughout human history are related to psychological trauma; this hypothesis could be tested in surviving indigenous cultures using the DES, the DDIS, the SCID-D, and the MID.

Trauma and Dissociation in the DSM-IV-TR

The inclusion of a dissociative disorders section in DSM-III in 1980 does not by itself prove the reliability or validity of the disorders in that section. However, the category and the five dissociative disorders within it have been retained in all subsequent editions up to DSM-IV-TR in 2000. The disorders, especially DID, had to survive a sustained attack on them in the popular media, the professional literature, and the courts during this time (Brown et al., 1998). No other disorders in the DSM were subjected to anything remotely approaching this degree of hostile attack.

In *State v. Greene* (cited in Scheflin, 2003), the Washington Supreme Court stated, DID is generally accepted within the scientific community as a diagnosable psychiatric condition" (p. 2). Similarly, in an opinion based on thirteen judicial opinions from state and federal courts, the West Virginia Supreme Court (*State v. Lockhart,* cited in Scheflin, 2003), found that numerous courts have allowed expert testimony on DID.

For expert scientific testimony to be allowed in a court of law, it must be based on a body of science that is accepted by the scientific community. Opposing counsel has the right to challenge this conclusion in a special hearing called a Frye or Daubert hearing, in which all arguments and evidence to the contrary can be presented; therefore, expert testimony about DID has survived the most rigorous legal challenges.

The inclusion of the dissociative disorders in the DSM-IV means that their validity has been accepted by the relevant scientific community, namely the American Psychiatric Association. In 1994, a new category of dissociative response to trauma was added to the DSM-IV—acute stress disorder, which includes traumatic amnesia among its diagnostic criteria. For new disorders to be included in DSM-IV, they had to be supported by a body of empirical data and they had to survive the critical review of several levels of committees— many of these levels and committee members were not particularly sympathetic to the dissociative disorders. Acute stress disorder was included in DSM-IV despite an overall political climate that was not highly receptive to the trauma-dissociation model.

The dissociative symptoms listed under Criterion B for acute stress disorder include "(3) derealization (4) depersonalization (5) dissociative amnesia (i.e., inability to recall an important aspect of the trauma)."

DSM-IV-TR symptoms of post-traumatic stress disorder include "dissociative flashback episodes" and "inability to recall an important aspect of the trauma."

Similarly, DSM-IV-TR dissociative amnesia Criterion A is "one or more episodes of inability to recall important personal information, usually of a traumatic or stressful nature, that is too extensive to be explained by ordinary forgetfulness."

One of the forms of DDNOS in DSM-IV-TR is "states of dissociation that occur in individuals who have been subjected to periods of prolonged and intense coercive persuasion (e.g., brainwashing, thought reform, or indoctrination while captive)."*

Thus, trauma-induced pathological dissociation is incorporated in the diagnostic criteria for four DSM-IV-TR disorders, plus DID, which by itself provides conclusive evidence that the existence of trauma-induced dissociation has been accepted by the relevant scientific community.

Surveys of Professional Opinion on Dissociation

Four surveys of professional opinion on the reliability and validity of the dissociative disorders, specifically including DID, have been conducted (Dunn et al., 1994; Lalonde et al., 2001; Mai, 1995; Pope et al., 1999). The only authors sympathetic to the validity of the dissociative disorders were Dunn et al. (1994). The other three surveys were conducted by authors who reject the validity of DID. These surveys, therefore, are not biased in favor of the dissociative disorders by the ideological positions of their authors.

---

*Reprinted with permission from the *Diagnostic and Statistical Manual of Mental Disorders,* Text Revision, pp. 468, 471, 523, 532. Copyright 2000. American Psychiatric Association.

Dunn et al. (1994) surveyed 1,120 Veterans Administration psychologists and psychiatrists and found that 97 percent believed in dissociative disorders and 80 percent in DID; 12.3 percent did not believe in DID; and 7.7 percent were unsure. Mai (1995) surveyed 180 Canadian psychiatrists and found that 66.1 percent believed in DID; 27.8 percent did not; and 3.3 percent were unsure. Of the 180 respondents, 56.7 percent had seen a case of DID; the average number of cases per psychiatrist was 3.78; and the average number of newly diagnosed cases per psychiatrist was 1.21.

Data from Pope et al. (1999) are discussed in Chapter 7. Lalonde et al. (2001) reported on responses to the same questionnaire by 403 Canadian psychiatrists. Out of the total 704 psychiatrists in the two surveys, 57 (8.1 percent) stated that dissociative amnesia should not be included in future editions of DSM, while 105 (14.9 percent) said that DID should not be included. Rejection of the validity of these two disorders is clearly an opinion of a small minority in psychiatry.

The number of psychiatrists who stated that there is partial or strong evidence for the validity of dissociative amnesia was 498 (70.7 percent); 144 (20.5 percent) said there was little evidence; and 61 (8.7 percent) had no opinion. For the number of psychiatrists stating that it has partial or strong validity was 470 (66.8 percent); 176 (25.0 percent) said there was little evidence; and 58 (8.2 percent) had no opinion. The existing opinion surveys strongly support the proposition that the validity of traumatic amnesia is accepted by the relevant scientific community, as is the validity of DID.

Peritraumatic Dissociation and Post-Traumatic Stress Disorder

The new DSM-IV category of acute stress disorder was originally named *brief reactive dissociative disorder*. It was initially presented to the DSM-IV dissociative disorders committee, of which I was a member, by David Spiegel and Robert Spitzer. The category was designed to identify individuals who had an acute reaction to a traumatic event characterized predominantly by dissociative symptoms (peritraumatic dissociation). The event and the reaction to it were too severe to be captured by the adjustment disorders, and they were not adequately described by any other criteria set in DSM-III-R.

After discussion and review, it was concluded that if the symptoms persisted beyond one month, the diagnosis would be changed to PTSD. This made sense, except for the problem that overnight an affected individual would switch from having a dissociative disorder to an anxiety disorder. To solve this problem, the new entity was renamed acute stress disorder and moved to the anxiety disorders section of DSM-IV. The criteria were then modified to follow the same format as PTSD, with the initial dissociative reaction retained among the B criteria for the disorder.

The dissociative and PTSD committee members unanimously voted in favor of PTSD, acute stress disorder, and the dissociative disorders all being included in a single trauma category; however, this recommendation was not accepted (the vote is itself evidence in favor of the trauma-dissociation model). As a result, we have in DSM-IV-TR an anxiety disorder, acute stress disorder, which was originally a dissociative disorder. This is not a practical problem for clinicians, but it illustrates the point that the DSM system does not handle psychological trauma very well. I have proposed organizational solutions to this problem in *The Trauma Model* (Ross, 2000b).

This history highlights a conceptual and scientific question: do acute dissociative reactions to trauma predict the later development of PTSD? The answer is yes, based on prospective studies of objectively verified trauma.

Koopman, Classen, and Spiegel (1994) studied reactions of 154 subjects to the 1991 Oakland/Berkeley firestorm. They measured dissociative symptoms with the Stanford Acute Stress Reaction Questionnaire, and 94 percent of the questionnaires were completed within three weeks of the fire. They conducted follow-up assessments with the Schedule of Recent Experience, Impact of Event Scale, and Civilian Version of the Mississippi Scale for Combat-Related Posttraumatic Stress Disorder; 87 percent of the follow-up questionnaires were received in the eighth month after the storm and 97 percent by the ninth month.

Of the 154 respondents, 57 percent had been evacuated from their homes and 22 percent lost their homes to the fire. Koopman, Classen, and Spiegel (1994) found that the best predictors of PTSD at follow-up on a regression analysis were dissociative symptoms at initial assessment (beta weight 0.26) and subsequent stressful events (beta weight 0.31).

The authors also reported on a set of Schneiderian symptoms embedded in the Stanford Acute Stress Reaction Questionaire within a scale measuring loss of personal autonomy. This scale had a moderate level of internal consistency as measured by a Cronbach's alpha of 0.63, and it predicted PTSD at a beta of 0.20. Thus, this study demonstrated two things: Schneiderian symptoms can be part of an acute response to objective severe trauma, and they can predict subsequent development of PTSD.

Koopman, Classen, and Spiegel (1996) undertook a further analysis of their Oakland/Berkeley firestorm data. They found that the number of dissociative symptoms increased among subjects who were more directly involved in the fire. Individuals with low contact endorsed an average of 3.0 dissociative symptoms; those with medium contact, 4.8; and those with high contact, 8.6 ($F = 12.30, p < .001$). The authors demonstrated a trauma-dissociation dose-response curve in reaction to a recent, severe, objective trauma. From my perspective, Schneiderian symptoms are a cluster of dissociative symptoms; Koopman, Classen, and Spiegel (1994, 1996) provide additional evidence that psychosis and dissociation are not discrete categories.

In five other studies reviewed by Koopman, Classen, and Spiegel (1994), dissociative symptoms were present in response to objective acute trauma including that experienced by New York emergency workers (Goldfarb, 1992) and victims of the Bay Area earthquake (Cardena and Spiegel, 1989), automobile accidents (Noyes et al., 1977), an ambush in Namibia (Feinstein, 1989), and a hostage-taking incident (Hillman, 1981). These five studies provide a body of evidence concerning objective trauma and overcome the methodological problem of retrospective reporting of trauma from decades earlier that limits the generalizability and validity of many studies with the DES, DDIS, and SCID-D.

More recently, Spiegel and Butler (2002) described symptoms of depression, PTSD, and dissociation following the terrorist attacks of September 11, 2001. Symptoms included depersonalization, derealization, and amnesia. Similarly, Silver et al. (2002) reported that 31.7 percent of 933 respondents to a nationwide survey reported dissociative symptoms nine to twenty-three days after September 11. They did not examine whether these dissociative symptoms predicted post-traumatic stress symptoms, which they observed at a high level in 17.0 percent of subjects at two months and 5.8 percent of subjects at six months.

Marmar et al. (1994) studied peritraumatic dissociation among Vietnam veterans on a retrospective basis using the DES and the Peritraumatic Dissociation Experiences Questionnaire. This study suffered from the limitation that reports of dissociation during combat were retrospective. However, they found significant correlations in the range of $r = 0.39$-0.60 between peritraumatic dissociation and a number of measures of PTSD and current DES scores. No such correlations were found for a wide range of other clinical scales on the MMPI-2; therefore the relationship between peritraumatic dissociation and later PTSD was specific. The ability of peritraumatic dissociation to predict later PTSD independently of combat exposure was demonstrated in a hierarchical logistic regression, providing further evidence in support of the trauma-dissociation model.

Fullerton et al. (2000) studied peritraumatic dissociation in 122 motor vehicle accident victims interviewed fourteen to twenty-one days after their accidents. They found that 79 percent of the subjects reported peritraumatic dissociation. The most common symptoms were that: the event seemed unreal as in a dream or play (39 percent) and moments of losing track or blanking out (32 percent). The significant predictors of peritraumatic dissociation in a hierarchical multiple regression were age, passenger injury, and prior major depression. These predictors point to the complex relationship between PTSD, peritraumatic dissociation, depression, and other forms of comorbidity.

Marmar et al. (1999) studied trauma exposure, peritraumatic dissociation, and PTSD in a prospective study of 322 rescue workers involved in the response to the Loma Prieta earthquake. They found that peritraumatic dissociation predicted later PTSD in a hierarchical regression analysis.

Morgan et al. (2001) studied peritraumatic dissociation among 155 military subjects exposed to the stress of military training. The soldiers completed the Clinician-Administered Dissociative States Scale in one of two studies reported by the authors. There were high levels of poststress dissociation in both studies. In the second study, measurements were taken before and after the stress and subjects were divided into general infantry soldiers (N = 41) and special forces soldiers (N = 18). Average dissociation scores for general infantry soldiers were 6.0 before exposure and 21.3 after exposure, whereas for special forces soldiers they were 1.6 before exposure and 9.7 after exposure, demonstrating that the special forces personnel were more stress resistant. The authors also found that previous exposure to a perceived threat to life increased both baseline and postexposure dissociation scales in both types of soldiers.

Other studies in which a significant relationship between peritraumatic dissociation and subsequent risk for PTSD was observed include Bernat et al. (1998); Maercker, Beauducel, and Schutzwohl (2000); Shalev et al. (1996); Kaufman et al. (2002); and Bremner and Brett (1997).

Additional studies demonstrating the occurrence of dissociation in response to trauma include Dancu et al. (1996); Feeny, Zoellner, and Foa (2000); Carlson et al. (2001); Zelikovsky and Lynn (2002); and Bremner, Krystal, et al. (1998). These references are illustrative but not exhaustive. Recent reviews of this literature include Bremner (2002) and Nijenhuis, van der Hart, and Steele (2002).

The literature on acute reactions to objectively verified trauma follows the pattern seen in studies of dissociative adults who report serious, chronic childhood trauma. The greater the trauma, the greater the degree of dissociation, and vice versa. Although much of the literature on trauma and dissociation involves current dissociation in adults who report unverified childhood trauma, the pattern among such subjects is the same as that observed in prospective studies of adult reactions to verified traumatic events.

Only two studies have involved systematic attempts to verify the childhood traumas reported by adults and adolescents in treatment for dissociative disorders (Coons, 1986, 1994). In one study (Coons, 1986), confirmation of abuse was obtained in seventeen out of twenty adult cases of DID, while in the other (Coons, 1994), confirmation was obtained in eighteen out of nineteen adolescent cases of DID and DDNOS. Since these are the only two studies of this type, I conclude, based on the existing data, that most trauma reports of DID and DDNOS are reasonably accurate. That conclusion is not reached lightly; I have discussed the problem of inaccurate or confabulated

trauma memories at length in previous writings on trauma and dissociation (Ross, 1995, 1997, 1999, 2000a,b).

There is an extensive clinical literature on dissociative fugue occurring in reaction to verified trauma, usually military combat. Dissociative fugue involves two of the core features of pathological dissociation
measured by the SCID-D (Steinberg, 1995): identity alteration and
amnesia. This literature supports the trauma-dissociation model and
provides clinical evidence of the occurrence of peritraumatic dissociation. Many of the fugue cases described in this literature were reported
over half a century ago (Fisher, 1945, 1947; Fisher and Joseph, 1949;
Loewenstein, 1993, 1996).

Trauma and Dissociation in Clinical Samples

In the first study comparing individuals with multiple personality
disorder (MPD) to people with other Axis I disorders, I administered
the DES and DDIS to twenty people with MPD, twenty with panic
disorder, twenty with eating disorders, and twenty with schizophrenia (Ross, Heber, Norton, and Anderson, 1989). Results of this study
are shown in Table 8.2.

This study demonstrated a pattern confirmed by all subsequent research: subjects with dissociative disorders report more dissociative
symptoms, more psychotic symptoms, and more trauma than do

TABLE 8.2. Trauma, dissociation, and psychosis in multiple personality disorder
(MPD), schizophrenia, panic disorder, and eating disorders

	MPD (N = 20)	Schizophrenia (N = 20)	Panic disorder (N = 20)	Eating disorders (N = 20)
Schneiderian* symptoms	6.6	4.4	0.3	1.7
Secondary* features of MPD	8.3	2.4	0.7	1.4
Sexual abuse	80%	10%	10%	20%
Physical abuse	75%	25%	5%	25%

Source: Adapted from Ross, Heber, Norton, and Anderson, 1989.

*Average number of symptoms per patient

those in other diagnostic groups (Carlson et al., 1993; Ross, 1997). For instance, in one study (Fink and Golinkoff, 1990) subjects with MPD reported more positive symptoms of schizophrenia than subjects with schizophrenia on MMPI Scales F and Sc and the Millon Clinical Multiaxial Inventory Scales named schizoid, schizotypal, thought disorder, and delusional disorder.

Five large case series shown in Table 8.3 confirm the high rates of childhood physical and sexual abuse in MPD (Coons, Bowman, and Milstein, 1988; Putnam et al., 1986; Ross, Miller, Reagor, et al., 1990; Ross, Norton, and Wozney, 1989; Schultz, Braun, and Kluft, 1989). Rates of physical and sexual abuse were reported in all five series, but in two the rate of physical and/or sexual abuse was not reported by the authors and could not be calculated from the published data. I include these two studies in Table 8.3 because they provide additional replication of the high rates of physical and sexual abuse in MPD, even though they do not provide data on the overall category of physical and/or sexual abuse.

The differences between MPD/DID and other diagnostic categories, in clinical experience and in the literature, include both higher rates of childhood physical and sexual abuse, and more severe abuse. Measures of severity embedded in the DDIS include age at onset of physical and sexual abuse; duration of physical and sexual abuse; frequency of physical and sexual abuse; number of types of sexual abuse perpetrated; and number of perpetrators of physical and sexual abuse. Other components of the severity of physical and sexual abuse not in-

TABLE 8.3. Rates of reported childhood physical and sexual abuse in five large series of multiple personality disorder cases (in percent)

	A (N = 100)	B (N = 50)	C (N = 236)	D (N = 355)	E (N = 102)
Sexual abuse	83.0	68.0	79.2	86.0	90.2
Physical abuse	75.0	60.0	74.9	82.0	82.4
Physical and/or sexual abuse	–	96.0	95.1	–	95.1

Note: A, Putnam et al., 1986; B, Coons, Bowman, and Milstein, 1988; C, Ross, Norton, and Wozney, 1989; D, Schultz, Braun, and Kluft, 1989; E, Ross, Miller, Reagor, et al., 1990

quired about by the DDIS include degree of coercion; combination with other forms of abuse and neglect; whether the perpetrator is a family member or stranger; degree of attachment to and dependency on the perpetrator; degree of bizarreness of the abuse; and witnessing the abuse of siblings or other children.

Most of these elements of severity have been quantified in empirical studies. An overall numerical measure of total trauma dose would, I predict, show more powerful correlations with degree of dissociation than the simple presence or absence of physical and sexual abuse. An excellent example of the quantification of physical and psychological abuse is the study by Zelikovsky and Lynn (2002), which confirms this prediction.

There are two ways to look at data such as that in Ross, Heber, Norton, and Anderson (1989). One is to conclude that MPD/DID is a more dissociative and trauma-related diagnostic category than schizophrenia, panic disorder, and eating disorders, which is true. Another way to examine the data, however, is to ask, How large is the trauma-dissociation subgroup within a given diagnostic category?

The size of the trauma-dissociation subgroup within DSM diagnostic categories should form a hierarchy; the trauma-dissociation subgroup is large in certain diagnostic categories, intermediate in others, and small or negligible in yet others. By definition, it constitutes 100 percent of DID. Based on clinical experience and my reading of the psychiatric literature, I predict that the hierarchy takes the form shown in Figure 8.1.

I predict that the size of the trauma-dissociation subgroup within schizophrenia is in the range of 25 to 40 percent of individuals who receive that diagnosis clinically. The empirical evidence supporting this prediction is reviewed in Chapter 11.

An additional prediction of my model is that the hierarchy shown in Figure 8.1 will closely resemble the hierarchy of comorbidity in DID (Ellason, Ross, and Fuchs, 1996). Generalized anxiety disorder is one of the most infrequent comorbid diagnoses in DID (frequency 1 percent), whereas PTSD has a frequency of 80 percent. The base rate of generalized anxiety disorder in the general population is 1 percent, while that of PTSD is about 7 percent. People with DID have higher rates of PTSD than the general population because they have correspondingly higher rates of trauma.

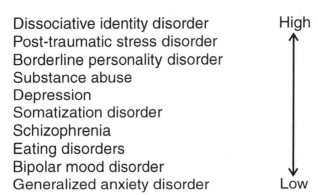

FIGURE 8.1. Size of the trauma-dissociation subgroup within DSM-IV-TR diagnostic categories (ranked from high to low)

This prediction is self-evident for PTSD, but it applies to all DSM diagnostic categories to some degree. In the case of generalized anxiety disorder, the trauma-dissociation subgroup may be no larger than it is in the general population overall; therefore, the degree to which the prediction applies may be zero. In schizophrenia, in comparison, the trauma-dissociation subgroup is an order of magnitude larger than it is in the general population, according to my model. This conclusion is based on the finding that about 3 percent of the general population is in the dissociative taxon (Waller and Ross, 1997), while 25 to 40 percent of people with schizophrenia meet criteria for a chronic, complex dissociative disorder (see Chapter 11).

The hierarchy of comorbidity in DID takes the form it does because it provides a measure of how trauma-related the various DSM categories are—disorders are more frequently comorbid in DID because they are more trauma related. Stated differently, a disorder highly comorbid with DID has a large trauma-dissociation subgroup.

According to my model, dissociative schizophrenia is as trauma related as DID. Similarly, the trauma-dissociation subgroup within eating disorders should have more trauma, comorbidity, psychobiology of trauma, and auditory hallucinations than the nontrauma subgroup (Vanderlinden and Vandereycken, 1997). Irrespective of their primary clinical diagnosis, individuals in the trauma-dissociation subgroup of different DSM categories should resemble one another and have the same treatment needs. I predict that they are more similar to one another than they are to nontrauma subjects within the same diagnostic category.

This thinking is similar to the model proposed by Bremner (2002), except that Bremner does not include schizophrenia within his spectrum of trauma disorders. Bremner's trauma disorder spectrum resembles the proposed DSM category disorder of extreme stress not otherwise specified (DESNOS), which was recently reviewed by Pain (2002). Epidemiological data on DESNOS demonstrate conclusively that it is the typical response to trauma, and that pure PTSD is relatively rare.

The basic idea of DESNOS is that DSM-IV-TR PTSD is only one component of the trauma response, which characteristically spans numerous DSM categories. My thesis is that psychosis is a characteristic element of the trauma response. Allen (2001) provides an approach to the problem of trauma, dissociation, and comorbidity that is consistent with the models of Bremner (2002) and Ross (2000b). Allen also provides a great deal of detail on therapy for the traumatized and highly comorbid individual.

Additional studies confirming the relationship between trauma and dissociation in clinical samples include Chu and Dill (1990), Waldinger et al. (1994), Carlson et al. (1993), and studies reviewed by Bremner (2002), Bremner and Marmar (1998), Nijenhuis (1992), Nijenhuis, van der Hart, and Steele (2002), Chu (1998), Vanderlinden (1993), and Ross (1997, 1999). The evidence for a relationship between trauma and dissociation in clinical populations is voluminous.

Trauma and Dissociation in Nonclinical Samples

Three surveys of trauma and dissociation in the general population have been undertaken: one in Canada (Ross, 1991), one in Turkey (Akyuz et al., 1999), and one in China (Ross, Keyes, and Xiao, 2002). Data from China are currently being analyzed; the study involved administration of the DES, PANSS, and DDIS to 424 general adult psychiatric inpatients, 304 general adult psychiatric outpatients, and 617 members of the general population.

Childhood physical abuse was reported by 13.2 percent of the outpatients, 5.4 percent of the inpatients, and 0.2 percent of the general population. Childhood sexual abuse was reported by 3.0 percent of the inpatients, 2.8 percent of the outpatients, and none of the general population subjects. Based on this survey, it appears that childhood physical and sexual abuse is much less common in China than in North America. However, when these abuses occur, they are significant risk factors for receiving psychiatric treatment as an adult.

In China, the same pattern was observed for dissociation: DES scores and the frequency of secondary features of DID were lower than in North America but higher in the clinical than nonclinical subjects. The overall conclusion is that the trauma-dissociation relationship appears to hold in China but affects a lower percentage of the population than in North America. More detailed analysis of these data will be reported in the future.

In the Turkish study (Akyuz et al., 1999) the DES was administered to 994 subjects in Sivas City. The DDIS was then administered to thirty-two subjects scoring above 17 on the DES and thirty-two matched subjects scoring under 10 on the DES. Of the high DES scorers, 53.1 percent met criteria for a dissociative disorder on the DDIS, compared to none of the low scorers. The authors inquired about physical and sexual abuse using the DDIS and also about neglect and emotional abuse; 65.6 percent of the high scorers reported one or more types of abuse compared to 28.1 percent of the low scorers (chi-square $= 9.04$, $p < .005$).

The minimum prevalence of DID in the general population of Turkey was determined to be 0.4 percent in this study, and the frequency of dissociative disorders including DID was 1.7 percent. The high DES scorers reported an average of 2.7 Schneiderian symptoms on the DDIS compared to 1.0 for the low scorers ($t = 2.87$, $p < .01$).

In contrast, in a general adult psychiatric inpatient sample in Turkey (Tutkun et al., 1998), the frequency of dissociative disorders was 14.5 percent, including 5.4 percent with DID. The average DES score among seventeen subjects with a DDIS dissociative disorder was 48.3; a matched group of nineteen subjects with no dissociative disorder on the DDIS had an average DES score of 5.0. The DDIS dissociative disorder group reported a frequency of childhood sexual and/or physical abuse of 82.4 percent compared to 26.3 percent for the nondissociative group (chi square $= 11.30$, $p < .001$). The DDIS dissociative disorder group reported an average of 6.4 Schneiderian symptoms compared to 1.6 for the nondissociative group.

In Turkey, then, trauma, dissociation, and positive symptoms of schizophrenia co-occur and the trauma-dissociation-psychosis group is much larger among psychiatric inpatients than in the general population.

In Winnipeg, Canada, the same pattern holds (Ross, 1991; Ross, Anderson, et al., 1991). In a stratified cluster sample of 454 subjects from the general population, the prevalence of dissociative disorders was 11.2 percent including 1.3 percent with MPD. According to the DDIS, the prevalence of DID was 3.1 percent, but I judged that most of these were false positives based on their DDIS profiles. These false-positive subjects did not report childhood physical or sexual abuse and had far fewer symptoms in the different sections of the DDIS than norms for DID (see DDIS norms for DID in Chapter 11). Their DDIS profiles were markedly different from norms for confirmed clinical cases of DID; these false-positive subjects did not belong to the category of severe, chronic, highly comorbid mental disorder.

Among subjects reporting childhood physical and/or sexual abuse, the prevalence of MPD on the DDIS was 10.5 percent compared to 2.0 percent for nonabused respondents. In a stepwise regression analysis with Schneiderian symptoms as the criterion variable, secondary features of MPD had a beta weight of 0.26 as a predictor, while physical and/or sexual abuse had a beta weight of 0.16. Data on Schneiderian symptoms from this study were reviewed in Chapter 6.

Among 299 general adult psychiatric inpatients in Winnipeg (Ross, Anderson, et al., 1991), the prevalence of dissociative disorders was 20.7 percent, including 5.4 percent with MPD. The three general population studies and the three psychiatric inpatient studies were conducted in distinct cultures and languages using the same measures, the DES and the DDIS, and therefore are directly comparable to one another.

Three studies of trauma and dissociation using the DES and DDIS have been conducted among college students as well—two in the United States (Murphy, 1994; Zelikovosky and Lynn, 2002) and one in Canada (Ross, Ryan, et al., 1991). In the Murphy study, I participated by making a rater judgment concerning whether DDIS profiles on selected subjects were true or false positives for dissociative disorders, but I was not otherwise involved in subject selection or data analysis. I had no involvement in the Zelikovsky and Lynn (2002) study.

A relationship between diagnosable dissociative disorders and trauma was found in all three studies. In the Ross, Ryan, et al. (1991) study, the DES was administered to 345 college undergraduates in Winnipeg; further measures were administered to 22 subjects scoring below 5 on the DES and 20 subjects scoring above 20 on the DES. The high-DES group had higher scores on all subscales of the SCL-90 including psychoticism (average score 2.04 versus 1.23, $p <$ .0001), and on fifteen out of twenty scales on the Millon Clinical Multiaxial Inventory-I, including schizoid, schizotypal, psychotic thinking, and psychotic delusions (all significant at $p < .007$ or less) (Ryan, 1988). The high-DES group reported an average of 4.4 Schneiderian symptoms on the DDIS, compared to 0.2 in the low group ($t = 5.190$, $p < .00001$).

Rates of sexual abuse were 35.0 percent in the high-DES group compared to 9.1 percent in the low-DES group. Rates of physical abuse were 35.0 percent in the high-DES group compared to 18.2 percent in the low-DES group. Based on extrapolation from the DDIS data, the prevalence of dissociative disorders among the 345 subjects was estimated to be 11.0 percent; among the high-DES group eight subjects were positive for MPD on the DDIS. The findings among college students, then, follow the same pattern as those in the general population.

The Psychobiology of Trauma and Dissociation

Reviews of the psychobiology of trauma and dissociation include Bremner (2002), Forrest (2001), Heim and Nemeroff (1999), Nijenhuis (1999), Nijenhuis, van der Hart, and Steele (2002), Krystal et al. (1998), and Zahn, Moraga, and Ray (1996). A number of different neurotransmitters and hormones including cortisol, endorphins, norepinephrine, neuropeptide Y, and glutamate are involved in the trauma response and pathological dissociation. The brain structures most directly involved in trauma and dissociation include the hippocampus, amygdala, thalamus, cingulate gyrus, insula, and medial prefrontal cortex.

Lanius, Williamson, and Menon (2002) reported that about 30 percent of subjects with PTSD exhibit a dissociative response to trauma imagery provocation studies. While reliving prior trauma in response to laboratory stimuli, for instance, about 70 percent of subjects show an increase in heart rate and 30 percent show a decrease. The dissociative subgroup of subjects exhibits higher levels of brain activation on fMRI (functional magnetic resonance imaging) in brain areas including the temporal and parietal lobes and the medial prefrontal cortex. The aroused, anxious, and nondissociative subjects, in contrast, show reduced activation in relevant areas of the brain. Such data provide evidence of brain circuitry that results in dissociation of physiology and psychology through active dampening of responses to stimuli.

The pathophysiology of trauma and dissociation are most recently and most thoroughly reviewed by Nijenhuis et al. (2002). I do not repeat their review in detail but highlight several interesting aspects of the pathophysiology.

One of the most active areas of investigation is the effect of cortisol on the hippocampus. Acute psychological trauma activates the hypothalamic-pituitary-adrenal (HPA) axis, resulting in elevated levels of serum cortisol (Sapolsky, 2000). However, chronic trauma may result in exhaustion or down-regulation of the HPA axis, with low levels of serum cortisol and blunted responses to challenges with corticotropin-releasing factor and adrenocorticotrophic hormone.

During the acute trauma response, high cortisol levels affect gating mechanisms in the cell walls of hippocampal neurons, resulting in entry of toxic metabolites into the neurons. These then cause damage and/or destruction of hippocampal neurons, as measured in laboratory mammals (Sapolsky, 2000).

A damaged hippocampus should fail to carry out its primary task, which is the integration of sensory, emotional, cognitive, and other input into coherent experiences and memories. Clinically, this should result in a failure of integration of memory, sensation, arousal, cognition, and identity—it should result in dissociation (Nijenhuis et al., 2002). Evidence for damage to the hippocampus due to psychological trauma is conclusive in laboratory mammals. MRI scans of samples of human subjects with PTSD due to combat and childhood sexual abuse suggest that the hippocampus may be smaller in individuals with PTSD than in normal controls (Stein et al., 1997).

In a study by Nijenhuis, Ehling, and Krikke (2002) the reduction in hippocampal volume in DID was 21 percent, which is by far the largest magnitude of any population studied to date. The task now is to replicate these findings, then to conduct prospective studies to determine whether hippocampal volume increases with response to treatment. An alternative possibility is that the subjects who reached integration had larger hippocampal volumes prior to therapy; in this case, larger volume would predict better treatment response, rather than functioning as a treatment outcome measure.

This line of investigation is new, and results are not yet conclusive for humans. However, the psychobiology of trauma and dissociation will be the focus of a great deal of research over the next decade. One can subject laboratory animals to severe, chronic psychological trauma and then study resulting dysregulations in the HPA axis and other biological systems. Causal attributions can be made in such studies using genetically homogeneous strains of experimental and control animals.

The ultimate goal is to demonstrate negative functional and structural biological impacts of trauma, then correction of the damage with medications and/or psychotherapy. The trauma model (Ross, 2000b) predicts that psychotherapy can initiate brain self-repair, resulting in neuronal regeneration in the hippocampus, and correction of faulty feedback and repair of other regulatory mechanisms perturbed by trauma. Similar effects can be obtained with medications, but the best results should be found with a combination of medication and psychotherapy. Symptoms treated with psychotherapy will include the positive symptoms of schizophrenia.

If these predictions prove to be correct, then the psychobiology of trauma and dissociation will become truly medical. Functional and structural brain imaging techniques will be utilized as treatment outcome measures in trials of psychotherapy, within this model, as will measures of HPA axis function. Another type of scan that might function as a psychotherapy outcome measure is proton magnetic resonance spectroscopy of N-acetyl-aspartate activity in the hippocampus (Villarreal et al., 2002). N-acetyl-aspartate activity levels should be low at the beginning of therapy and should normalize with recovery, if the model is correct.

Given the present state of technology and knowledge of the biology of trauma, such studies can be undertaken in this decade. They were impossible fifteen years ago because we did not have adequate symptom measures, had not sketched in the psychobiology of trauma to a sufficient degree, and had no conceptual model for such a program of research. The psychobiology of trauma and dissociation is one of the most interesting and promising areas in biological psychiatry. It has the potential to provide conclusive evidence for the trauma-dissociation model.

Chapter 9

Dissociative Identity Disorder

In this chapter, I briefly review the reliability, validity, etiology, epidemiology, and phenomenology of dissociative identity disorder. More comprehensive reviews are available in Cohen, Berzoff, and Elin (1995), Michelson and Ray (1996), Ross (1997), and other sources discussed in Chapter 7. My purpose is to outline a literature unfamiliar to most clinicians, researchers, and laypeople interested in schizophrenia. I realize that this chapter falls far short of a comprehensive review. However, my aim here is to establish that there is a replicated body of findings concerning DID.

The scientific literature on chronic, complex dissociation provides a foundation for the dissociative subtype of schizophrenia. This literature did not exist before the mid-1970s. Bleuler (1950 [1911]) described dissociative schizophrenia in great detail nearly a century ago (see Chapter 10), but no valid and reliable measures of dissociation were available for him to use. A scientifically testable theory of dissociative schizophrenia required two developments, the first of which was the publication of the DSM-III in 1980 by the American Psychiatric Association. The DSM-III provided operationalized diagnostic criteria that could be subjected to formal studies of reliability and validity.

The second development was the inauguration of a scientific literature on measurement of pathological dissociation, which occurred with Bernstein and Putnam's (1986) publication of the DES. Eighteen years later, the psychometric literature on pathological dissociation has developed to a level that detailed, specific, testable predictions can be made about the relationships between trauma, dissociation, psychosis, and a broad range of comorbidity. In my brief review of this literature, I first examine data on the reliability and validity of DID.

The reliability and validity of DID have been demonstrated primarily by studies with the DES, DDIS, SCID-D, and the MDIS. Although the reliability, or lack of reliability, of any DSM-IV-TR disorder can be demonstrated only through formal studies of interrater agreement, validity is a more complex concept. Many levels of evidence can contribute to validity including case studies, historical and anthropological data, physiological studies, and studies of concurrent validity.

Although in theory the dissociative subtype of schizophrenia could be valid and reliable independently of DID, in practice this is unlikely because the two disorders overlap so much phenomenologically. What is true of one is likely to be true of the other. If DID were to be reclassified as the dissociative subtype of schizophrenia, then it would be impossible for many cases of dissociative schizophrenia to be valid in the absence of validity for DID, by definition.

RELIABILITY AND VALIDITY

Consistent Phenomenology of Dissociative Identity Disorder

The phenomenology of DID was described in two large case series published in the 1980s (Putnam et al., 1986 [N = 100]; Ross, Norton, and Wozney, 1989 [N = 236]). These two reports were based on questionnaires completed by clinicians in mail-out surveys. Although the questionnaires, which were developed independently, had no reliability or formal validity, the two studies elevated the literature above the level of single cases and small series.

The two series were remarkably consistent on a large number of variables including types and frequencies of alter personalities, comorbidity, trauma histories, and treatment histories (Ross, 1997). They were also consistent with, and in fact based on, previous checklists and the single-case literature. In one series (N = 236), 40.8 percent of cases had a prior diagnosis of schizophrenia and 54.5 percent had been treated with antipsychotic medication; in the other series (N = 100), just under 50 percent of subjects had a prior diagnosis of schizophrenia.

Since those two initial large series, structured interview or systematic clinical profiles of DID have been accumulated in eight languages in ten countries, as shown in Table 9.1. The phenomenology of DID has remained consistent across all these studies, which is evidence for the reliability and validity of the disorder. For instance, in a series of 102 cases interviewed with the DDIS (Ross, Miller, Reagor, et al., 1990), 26.5 percent of subjects had a prior diagnosis of schizophrenia and 55.9 percent had been treated with antipsychotic medication.

The clinical profile of DID is consistent across different languages, cultures, and methodologies of data collection including individual case histories, mail-out questionnaires, and valid self-report measures and structured interviews. The heterogeneity of these sources of information provides evidence of validity because the findings arise from disparate tools and settings, and therefore cannot be artifacts of any one methodology.

Reliability of Dissociative Identity Disorder

The reliability of DID was initially established in studies using the DDIS (Ross, 1997; Ross, Heber, Norton, Anderson, Anderson, et al., 1989) and SCID-D (Steinberg, 1995; Steinberg, Rounsaville, and Cicchetti, 1990). A recent study (Ross, Duffy, and Ellason, 2002)

TABLE 9.1. Countries in which structured interview or clinical profiles of dissociative disorder cases have been gathered by investigators familiar with the modern literature

Country	Language	Structured interview
Canada	English	DDIS
United States	English	DDIS, SCID-D
Australia	English	DDIS
Norway	Norwegian	SCID-D
Netherlands	Dutch	SCID-D
Turkey	Turkish	DDIS, SCID-D
China	Chinese	DDIS
Puerto Rico	Spanish	Clinical
Germany	German	SCID-D
Japan	Japanese	DDIS

Note: The DDIS has also been translated into French, Italian, Polish, Ukranian, Hebrew, and Japanese.

provides the first information concerning the rates of agreement between DDIS, SCID-D, DES-T, and a clinician conducting a clinical interview.

In this study, we administered the DDIS and DES-T to a sample of 201 general adult psychiatric inpatients; a second interviewer blind to the results of the DDIS and DES-T then administered the SCID-D to 110 of these subjects. In the third stage of the study, the author who administered the SCID-D assigned fifty-two cases to me to interview clinically. These were an assortment of cases positive and negative for dissociative disorders on the DDIS and SCID-D, and I was blind to results of the first two interviews.

We found good rates of agreement on membership in the dissociative taxon, where taxon membership was defined in one of four ways: as a score above 20 on the DES-T; or as meeting criteria for DID or DDNOS on the DDIS, on the SCID-D, or on clinical interview. These results are shown in Box 9.1.

These rates of interrater agreement using Cohen's kappa are equivalent to those for schizophrenia, depression, substance abuse, and other Axis I categories. They provide evidence of concurrent validity, because the DES-T, DDIS, and SCID-D all have independently established reliability and validity (Pincus et al., 2000). The combined

---

BOX 9.1. Reliability of the dissociative disorders in an inpatient setting (Cohen's kappa): dissociative identity disorder or dissociative disorder not otherwise specified versus no dissociative disorder (N = 52)

DDIS–SCID-D	DDIS–Clinician	SCID-D–Clinician
0.74	0.71	0.56

DDIS–DES-T	SCID-D–DES-T	Clinician–DES-T
0.81	0.76	0.74

DDIS = Dissociative Disorders Interview Schedule; SCID-D = Structured Clinical Interview for DSM-IV Dissociative Disorders; DES-T = Taxometric Subscale of the Dissociative Experiences Scale

Source: Ross, Duffy, and Ellason, 2002. Reproduced by permission of The Haworth Maltreatment and Trauma Press.

category of DID and DDIS captures most cases of chronic, complex, pathological dissociation.

Although the quantity of literature on the reliability and validity of chronic, complex dissociation is small compared to that for schizophrenia and depression, that which exists is of adequate methodology. I predict, based on this literature, that the dissociative subtype of schizophrenia will be shown to have good reliability and validity, once its diagnostic criteria have been subjected to systematic studies.

The validity of pathological dissociation does not, in and of itself, prove anything about the dissociative subtype of schizophrenia. However, it provides a psychometric foundation for testing the reliability and validity of the proposed subtype. Valid and reliable measures of pathological dissociation are available in the literature early in the twenty-first century. That is why the dissociative subtype of schizophrenia is a testable scientific hypothesis. The fact that the reliability and validity of DID have been demonstrated proves that the same can be done for dissociative schizophrenia.

ETIOLOGY

The clinical and research literatures on DID provide overwhelming evidence for the traumatic origins of the disorder (Chu, 1998; Putnam, 1989; Ross, 1997) (see Table 8.2). However, an adequate etiological model for DID should be as complex and multifactorial as that for dissociative schizophrenia. Numerous influences affect the clinical picture, many of them not usually thought of as "trauma" (Loewenstein, 2002). These include verbal abuse and family rules, dynamics, and transactional patterns, for instance.

Worldwide, chronic childhood trauma is caused in large part by war, famine, disease, high infant mortality, and natural disasters. In North America these forms of trauma are less common. Therefore, in North America we tend to focus more on sexual abuse, physical abuse, neglect, and family violence as the main forms of childhood trauma.

The etiological models proposed by specialists in DID in the 1980s (Braun, 1986; Kluft, 1984; Putnam, 1989; Ross, 1989) are still accepted in the dissociative disorders field. They are exemplified by

Kluft's (1984) four-factor model. According to Kluft, DID is the out-come of a complex interaction between an innate ability to dissociate, childhood trauma, healing and restorative experiences that counter the effects of the trauma, and a host of other factors that affect devel-opment in all human beings. Kluft gives specific examples of healing and restorative experiences and discusses some of the nuances of how the four factors interact. His etiological model of DID is similar to the one for dissociative schizophrenia outlined in Chapter 1.

In clinical practice, I have never seen an inpatient case of DID in a person who did not experience a profoundly disturbed and traumatic childhood. Nor have I ever heard such a case described clinically, at a conference presentation, or in the written literature. The percentage of inpatients with DID who have experienced relatively normal child-hoods, in my clinical experience, is definitely less than 0.1 percent; it is probably at least several orders of magnitude lower than that, if not zero. For all practical purposes, inpatient DID is always a complex trauma disorder (Bremner, 2002).

As for any disorder, milder variants are encountered in the general population. The milder variants I have encountered clinically include much less severe comorbidity, much simpler personality systems, and much greater ease of treatment. For example, one woman in her twenties reported sexual abuse by a baby-sitter between ages eleven and thirteen that did not involve intercourse. She had one alter person-ality with whom she was almost fully coconscious, and she accepted the fact that the alter personality was a part of her without difficulty. Complex inpatient cases, in comparison, often resist accepting the fact that their alter personalities are parts of themselves.

Within the inpatient setting, there is also a gradient of severity of cases. When interviewing previously undiagnosed cases of DID on a general adult unit (Ross, Duffy, and Ellason, 2002), I saw simpler personality systems than I do in my trauma program. Patients are re-ferred to the trauma program by specialists in dissociative disorders and with DID diagnoses already made; they often have ten or more alter personalities with distinct names, ages, and functions.

The previously undiagnosed patients on the general adult unit, in comparison, usually had only three or four personality states. Besides the host personality, there was usually a traumatized child, an angry adolescent, and often a part that acted out sexually. The parts often did not have separate first names and were referred to as "The Angry Me," "Her," "The Other Me," or by some similar term. They could be categorized as child, adolescent, or adult but usually did not have specific ages. The patients came from less extremely dysfunctional family backgrounds than those in the trauma program. However, it is likely that the trauma histories and inventories of alter personalities were more extensive than I was able to determine in a single research interview with the general adult patients, so the gap between the general adult and trauma program cases is probably not as big as it seems.

There is controversy about the relative contributions of childhood trauma, iatrogenesis, and factitious disorder to cases of DID treated by specialists in North America (Loewenstein, 2002; Piper, 1997; Ross, 1997; Spanos, 1996). However, this controversy is at most marginally relevant to the dissociative subtype of schizophrenia. According to my theory, its etiology is primarily environmental and psychosocial in nature; positive symptoms of schizophrenia in the dissociative subtype have psychological meaning and function, and can be treated to stable remission with psychotherapy.

The trauma model of DID has both adherents and skeptics (see Chapter 7). All parties, however, are agreed that DID is a reaction to the environment. No one has proposed that DID is a biomedical disease, claimed that it has a specific endogenous biological cause, or suggested that it is inherited. Whether a person sees DID as an iatrogenic artifact or a naturally occurring response to childhood trauma, or a mixture of both, does not change the point of fundamental agreement: DID is a way that some but not all individuals react to certain types of environment.

To my knowledge, all investigators who have published data on clinical cases of DID adhere to the trauma model of DID. Psychiatrists who reject the validity of DID, such as Merskey (1995), McHugh (1997), and Piper (1997) have provided no data of their own on etiology, phenomenology, reliability, validity, or epidemiology. They have provided no operationalized alternative treatment plan for the population, and no treatment outcome or follow-up data of their own. The trauma model of DID, in comparison, is supported by empirical literature from many different countries.

If a substantial number of individuals with the dissociative subtype of schizophrenia also meet DSM-IV-TR criteria for DID or DDNOS, if the symptoms of schizophrenia and DID/DDNOS overlap extensively, and if it is agreed that the etiology of DID is primarily environmental, then it follows that the etiology of dissociative schizophrenia may be environmental. This argument provides limited support for the theory of a dissociative subtype of schizophrenia.

EPIDEMIOLOGY

If DID is rare, and if many individuals with dissociative schizophrenia also meet criteria for DID or DDNOS, then dissociative schizophrenia should also be rare. Conversely, if DID and DDNOS are relatively common among psychiatric inpatients, then it is more likely that dissociative schizophrenia is common. As I have been arguing throughout this book, this is not simply a matter of comorbidity. The phenomenology of DID and dissociative schizophrenia are to a large extent the same thing; that is why structured interviews make misdiagnoses in both directions. It is why many people in treatment for DID have prior diagnoses of schizophrenia.

DID and dissociative schizophrenia are not separate categories. They overlap a great deal. As I have proposed, there are several possible nosological solutions to this problem, but I am less invested in nosological solutions than I am in getting the problem acknowledged. If the problem does not exist, as it does not for the schizophrenia field up to this point, then there is nothing to discuss and no need for a solution.

Eleven studies in seven countries now provide data on the prevalence of undiagnosed DID and dissociative disorders among general adult psychiatric inpatients (Friedl and Draijer, 2000; Gast et al., 2001; Horen, Leichner, and Lawson, 1995; Knudsen et al., 1995; Latz, Kramer, and Hughes, 1995; Modestin et al., 1996; Rifkin et al., 1998; Ross, Anderson, et al., 1991; Ross, Keyes, and Xiao, 2002; Saxe et al., 1993; Tutkun et al., 1998). These studies were done in six languages on three continents. I will soon be adding data from China to the ten studies shown in Table 9.2 (Ross, Keyes, and Xiao, 2002). All the studies in Table 9.2 involved screening inpatients with the DES and then interviewing a group of high scorers with the DDIS or SCID-D.

TABLE 9.2. Prevalence of dissociative identity disorder and the dissociative disorders in inpatient settings in seven countries

Study	DID (%)	Dissociative disorder (%)	Structured interview
United States			
Ross, Duffy, Ellason, 2002 (N = 201)	7.5	40.8	DDIS
Rifkin et al., 1998 (N = 100)	1.0	n/a	SCID-D
Latz, Kramer, and Hughes 1995 (N = 175)	12.0	46.0	DDIS
Saxe, et al., 1993 (N = 110)	3.6	15.0	DDIS
Canada			
Horen, Leichner, and Lawson, 1995 (N = 48)	6.0	17.0	
Ross, Anderson, et al., 1991 (N = 299)	3.3	20.7	DDIS
Turkey			
Tutkun et al., 1998 (N = 166)	5.4	10.2	DDIS
Switzerland			
Modestin et al., 1996 (N = 207)	0.4	5.0	DDIS
Norway			
Knudsen et al., 1995 (N = 101)	4.9	7.9	SCID-D
Netherlands			
Friedl and Draijer, 2000 (N = 122)	1.7	8.2	SCID-D
Germany			
Gast et al., 2001 (N = 115)	0.9	4.3	SCID-D
Total (N = 1,644)	3.7	15.3	

Source: Adapted from Ross, Duffy, and Ellason, 2002.

Note: DDIS = Dissociative Disorders Interview Schedule; SCID-D = Structured Clinical Interview for DSM-IV

On average, undiagnosed DID affects 3.7 percent of general adult psychiatric inpatients, and 15.3 percent have some type of dissociative disorder. Since there are probably undetected cases of DID among the subjects with other dissociative disorders, it is reasonable to conclude that undiagnosed DID affects at least one out of every twenty-five general adult psychiatric inpatients. A complex, chronic dissociative disorder of some type affects about one in ten, possibly as many as one in six. Given the high degree of overlap between DID/DDNOS and schizophrenia (see Chapter 11), I conclude that dissociative schizohrenia is not rare among psychiatric inpatients.

Dissociative schizophrenia may affect 5 to 10 percent of general adult psychiatric inpatients. This estimate is based on three facts: 10 to 15 percent of psychiatric inpatients have chronic, complex dissociative disorders; 25 to 50 percent of individuals in treatment for DID have prior clinical diagnoses of schizophrenia; and two-thirds of individuals with clinical diagnoses of DID meet structured interview criteria for schizophrenia or schizoaffective disorder. The arithmetic is 5 percent (0.1×0.5) as a low-end estimate or 10 percent (0.15×0.67) as a high-end estimate.

My purpose is to establish a preliminary range for the frequency of dissociative schiophrenia among general adult psychiatric inpatients. It is not to provide a comprehensive review of the literature on the epidemiology of DID.

There are three studies of the prevalence of DID in the general population (Akyuz et al., 1999; Ross, 1991; Ross, Keyes, and Xiao, 2002), one each from Turkey, Canada, and China. All three studies used the DES and DDIS. The prevalence of DID in the general population is in the range of 0.4 to 1.3 percent according to these studies, which is very similar to the worldwide lifetime prevalence for schizophrenia of 1 percent. The point and lifetime prevalences of DID among adults should be the same, or very similar, since very few if any cases arise in adulthood.

If DID affected only one person in 10,000 in the general population, the overlap between DID and schizophrenia would occur in one person in a million, if they were independent disorders. Even if every case of DID was also a case of dissociative schizophrenia, dissociative schizophrenia would affect only one person in 10,000, or 1 percent of people with schizophrenia. For the theory of dissociative schizophrenia to be scientifically serious, DID must be about as common as schizophrenia; it cannot have a prevalence that is lower by two orders of magnitude. All the existing epidemiological data support the conclusion that DID is prevalent enough that it could commonly co-occur with schizophrenia.

If we assume that 3 percent of the population is in the dissociative taxon, as indicated by the DES-T data of Waller and Ross (1997), and if we assume that the lifetime prevalence of schizophrenia is 1 percent, then the prediction that dissociative schizophrenia affects 25 to 40 percent of individuals with schizophrenia means that only about 8 to 13 percent of people in the dissociative taxon have dissociative schizophrenia. The others have pathological dissociation but not schizophrenia. I mention these numbers to demonstrate that, based on the existing epidemiological data on pathological dissociation, the prediction that dissociative schizophrenia affects 0.25 to 0.4 percent of the population is arithmetically plausible.

Among individuals in treatment for chemical dependency problems, according to the four existing studies with the DES and DDIS totaling 401 subjects (Dunn, Paolo, Ryan, and Van Fleet 1994; Ellason et al., 1996; Leeper, Page, and Hendricks, 1992; Ross et al., 1992), undiagnosed DID affects 11.2 percent and dissociative disorders 31.7 percent. Therefore the dissociative subtype of schizophrenia may be more common among other clinical populations than it is among general adult psychiatric inpatients.

Table 9.3 shows the frequency of the different dissociative disorders in an inpatient setting according to the DDIS, SCID-D, and a clinician (myself) (Ross, Duffy, and Ellason, 2002). I include these data here because they demonstrate that, in this study, the most conservative diagnostician was the clinician. Given these findings, it is reasonable to use a prevalence of chronic complex dissociative disorders among psychiatric inpatients of 10 to 15 percent when estimating the prevalence of dissociative schizophrenia among general adult psychiatric inpatients.

The data from Ross, Duffy and Ellason (2002) are also consistent with my prediction that dissociative schizophrenia affects 25 to 40 percent of individuals in treatment for schizophrenia. This is the range for undiagnosed dissociative disorders among general adult inpatients in Ross, Duffy, and Ellason (2002), but it is higher than the

TABLE 9.3. Lifetime prevalence of the dissociative disorders according to three diagnostic methods in an inpatient setting (in percent)

Disorder	DDIS (N = 201)	SCID-D (N = 110)	Clinician (N = 52)
Dissociative amnesia	13.4	7.3	11.5
Dissociative fugue	0.0	0.0	0.0
Depersonalization disorder	4.5	8.2	1.9
Dissociative identity disorder	7.5	9.1	9.6
Dissociative disorder NOS	15.4	20.0	5.8
Some type of dissociative disorder	40.8	44.5	26.9

Source: Ross, Duffy, and Ellason, 2002. Reproduced by permission of The Haworth Maltreatment and Trauma Press.

average for the eleven international studies. I predict, then, that dissociative disorders, and hence the dissociative subtype of schizophrenia, are more common among individuals in treatment for schizophrenia than among general adult psychiatric inpatients. Data supporting this conclusion are presented in Chapter 11.

These calculations are intended to establish an estimate for the prevalence of dissociative schizophrenia, and to provide a set of arguments that the theory should be taken seriously on epidemiological grounds. Such estimates are a necessary foundation for the investment of significant research resources in studies of dissociative schizophrenia.

PHENOMENOLOGY

The phenomenology of DID was well described by Bleuler in his (1950 [1911]) text *Dementia Praecox or the Group of Schizophrenias*. It is also described in detail in Putnam (1989), Ross (1989, 1997), and in extensive literature cited in those references (see also Ross, 1994; 1995). I discuss the positive symptoms of schizophrenia in DID at length in Chapter 11, and so review them only briefly here.

Two early large case series of MPD (Putnam et al., 1986; Ross, Norton, and Wozney, 1989) tabulated the trauma histories, treatment histories, details of the personality system, dissociative symptoms, and nondissociative comorbidity of MPD/DID. Subsequent studies have replicated these findings with more refined methodology, just as these two series advanced the methodological status of the prior clinical literature.

In Ross, Norton, and Wozney (1989) 94.9 percent of 236 subjects endorsed amnesia between alter personalities. Because 100 percent endorsed the two DSM-III-R criteria for MPD, and because these are equivalent to the first two DSM-IV-TR criteria for DID, one can assume that the data on MPD are representative of DSM-IV-TR DID.

Of the 236 subjects, 63.7 percent had received a prior diagnosis of depression and 68.9 percent had been treated with antidepressants; 40.8 percent had received a prior diagnosis of schizophrenia and 54.5 percent had received antipsychotic medication. The average number of Schneiderian symptoms per subject was 4.5. These data led me to predict that a large percentage of DID subjects would meet criteria for schizophrenia or schizoaffective disorder on structured interview.

This prediction was confirmed in a later study using the Structured Clinical Interview for DSM-III-R (SCID) (Ellason, Ross, and Fuchs, 1996), in which 49.5 percent of 107 DID subjects met criteria for schizoaffective disorder, 18.7 percent for schizophrenia, and 74.3 percent for some type of psychotic disorder.

The high levels of comorbidity in DID span all of Axis I and II using the SCID, the Millon Clinical Multiaxial Inventory (Ellason and Ross, 1996), the Hopkins Symptom Checklist-90 (SCL-90) (Ellason and Ross, 1997b), and the MMPI (Armstrong, 1991; Armstrong and Loewenstein, 1990; Coons and Sterne, 1986).

In the study by Ellason, Ross, and Fuchs (1996), among 107 subjects with DID, comorbid depression was present in 97.2 percent, PTSD in 79.2 percent, panic disorder in 69.2 percent, substance abuse in 65.4 percent, obsessive-compulsive disorder in 63.6 percent, a somatoform disorder in 43.9 percent, and an eating disorder in 38.3 percent. On Axis II, 56.3 percent of 103 subjects met criteria for borderline personality disorder and 48.5 percent for avoidant personality disorder.

The average number of lifetime Axis I diagnoses per subject was 7.3 and the average number of personality disorders was 3.6, making a total of 10.9 psychiatric disorders. Since the SCID does not diagnose sleep disorders, psychosexual disorders, or dissociative disorders, all of which are nearly universal in inpatient DID, addition of these disorders would make a grand total of fourteen lifetime psychiatric diagnoses. These data are the foundation for the prediction that dissociative schizophrenia is characterized by extensive comorbidity on Axis I and II. A solution to the clinical, logical, and scientific conundrum presented by this level of comorbidity is presented in my book *The Trauma Model: A Solution to the Problem of Comorbidity in Psychiatry* (Ross, 2000b).

The DDIS (Ross, 1997) contains a section called Secondary Features of Dissociative Identity Disorder. If one imagined that there were separate people living inside the person with DID and further assumed that there were various combinations of types of amnesia between these people, then the secondary features would follow logically from switching of executive control. The Schneiderian symptoms follow logically from internal intrusions and communications between alter personalities.

The frequency of the sixteen secondary features of DID among 102 subjects with DID are shown in Table 9.4 (Ross, Miller, Reagor, et al., 1990). In this study, conducted in Winnipeg, Ottawa, California, and Utah, only the fifteen subjects from Ottawa were in treatment for DID; all the others completed the DDIS at the time of their initial diagnostic assessment for a dissociative disorder. Therefore, the data cannot be an artifact of treatment for DID. The full text of the DDIS is available in Ross (1997) and at <www.rossinst.com>.

These symptoms should also be characteristic of dissociative schizophrenia. I predict that they are an order of magnitude less common in the nondissociative subtypes of schizophrenia. The secondary features of DID, I predict, can discriminate the dissociative and non-dissociative subtypes of schizophrenia using statistical procedures ranging from simple comparisons of the average number of symptoms in each category to discriminant function analysis.

TABLE 9.4. Frequency of the secondary features of dissociative identity disorder (N = 102)

Item	Percent
Another person existing inside	90.2
Voices talking	87.3
Voices coming from inside	82.4
Another person taking control	81.4
Amnesia for childhood	81.4
Referring to oneself as "we" or "us"	73.5
Person inside has a different name	70.6
Blank spells	67.7
Flashbacks	66.7
Being told by others of unremembered events	62.8
Feelings of unreality	56.9
Strangers know the patient	44.1
Noticing that objects are missing	42.2
Coming out of blank spells in a strange place	36.3
Objects are present that cannot be accounted for	31.4
Different handwriting styles	27.5

Source: Ross, C. A., Miller, S. D., Reagor, R., et al., 1990, Figure 5, Table 3. *American Journal of Psychiatry,* 147, 596-601, 1990. Copyright 1990, the American Psychiatric Association; http://AJP.psychiatryonline.org. Reprinted by permission.

PART IV:
DISSOCIATIVE IDENTITY DISORDER AND SCHIZOPHRENIA

Chapter 10

Bleuler's Description of Schizophrenia

The purpose of this chapter is to establish several things: the dissociative subtype of schizophrenia is described in minute detail in Bleuler's classic 1911 text, *Dementia Praecox or the Group of Schizophrenias,* which was translated into English in 1950; dissociation was the fundamental phenomenon in Bleuler's schizophrenia; Bleuler's stature as a grandfather of the schizophrenia field has persisted while his description of schizophrenia has been forgotten; and an erroneous dichotomy between multiple personality disorder and schizophrenia has persisted in psychiatry since 1911. I believe that the evidence supporting these opinions is overwhelming.

Bleuler (1950 [1911]) is widely recognized as one of the leading authorities on schizophrenia of the entire twentieth century. Three of his four subtypes of schizophrenia appear in DSM-IV-TR—paranoid, catatonic, and undifferentiated, also known as hebephrenic. His fourth subtype, simple schizophrenia, corresponds to the DSM-IV-TR Cluster A personality disorders, paranoid, schizoid, and schizotypal.

Bleuler is known for his careful, detailed description of the phenomenology of schizophrenia. For instance, Kantor and Herron (1966), write that, "the descriptive accuracy of the Bleulerian 'signs' has led to their inclusion as an operational definition of schizophrenia in a recent psychiatric dictionary . . . the Bleulerian conception differs little from the official nomenclature of the American Psychiatric Association" (p. 9).

Gottesman (1991) states,

> Kraepelin and Bleuler provided detailed phenomenological sketches of dementia praecox/schizophrenia. Their sketches were strong on the descriptive psychopathology of the syndrome . . . Bleuler's reconceptualization contributed greatly to

the scientific understanding of schizophrenia as a disruption of the thought processes and feelings of persons who, in most other ways, are like ourselves. An unintended side effect of his term, however, was that many people came to believe that schizophrenics display multiple, or split, personalities. They do not. (p. 8)

In a similar vein, Torrey et al. (1994) state, "The popular but incorrect image of schizophrenia as a 'split personality' also reflects a belief that schizophrenia changes the personality, even splitting it into separate parts" (p. 144).

Besides coining the term *schizophrenia* and his careful phenomenology, Bleuler is also remembered for his "four As" of schizophrenia: ambivalence, autism, associations, and affect. According to Bleuler, the four As are all secondary to the core phenomenon in schizophrenia, which is a splitting or dissociation of mental contents. His name for the disorder, derived from the Greek, means "split-mind disorder." He chose the term because it captured the core of the phenomenology.

Contemporary commentators account for Bleuler's choice of the term *schizophrenia,* which he coined to replace Kraepelin's earlier term, *dementia praecox,* by saying that he had in mind either a split between thought and feeling or between reality and nonreality (see Chapter 11). These commentators fail to grasp the pervasive and fundamental role of splitting in Bleuler's schizophrenia.

Blueler is acknowledged as one of the great phenomenologists of schizophrenia, but most of his phenomenology has been forgotten. His description of schizophrenia is identical to contemporary descriptions of DID, if one excludes the cases with florid thought disorder. The role of splitting in Blueler's schizophrenia is identical to the role of dissociation in contemporary DID. Indeed, in Bleuler the two terms *splitting* and *dissociation* are synonyms.

I could travel back in time, walk into Bleuler's hospital in Zurich, Switzerland, the Burgholzli, and, except for the language barrier, treat a large number of his patients for DID. Bleuler's 1911 text provides an explicit, rich, and detailed portrait of DID, including its comorbidity. The text contains conclusive proof that DID was common among hospitalized mental patients in Switzerland early in the twentieth century. Bleuler was intimately familiar with the dissociative subtype of schizophrenia.

The myth that Bleuler's schizophrenia is entirely different from split or multiple personality has been accepted throughout psychiatry. The myth is so powerful and unquestioned that it has been accepted by psychiatrists, patients, and the general public. For example, Ian Chovil, writing on his Web page, <www.chovil.com>, about his own experience of schizophrenia, says, "Bleuler coined the term 'the schizophrenias,' meaning literally 'split mind,'—not to be confused with split personality, which is entirely different."

In his description of his own schizophrenia, however, Chovil states,

> My mind seemed to be falling apart into the left brain, me, and a right brain I hardly knew who was in tremendous pain and very demanding, and a dinosaur or core brain, very powerful and very angry at me.

One could not ask for a clearer description of dissociation of the personality within schizophrenia. Chovil's (2000) account of his illness in the *Schizophrenia Bulletin* is of particular interest because, by his description, he may have a nondissociative subtype of schizophrenia. If this is correct, then dissociation of the personality can be a major element of a schizophrenia not otherwise characterized by overt dissociative symptomatology. At a process level, Bleuler may be correct that dissociation is fundamental even in paranoid, catatonic, and hebephrenic schizophrenia.

ANALYSIS OF BLEULER'S 1911 TEXT ON SCHIZOPHRENIA

Origin of the Term Schizophrenia

Bleuler's explanation for his choice of the term *schizophrenia* bears quotation. Subsequent quotations will demonstrate the pervasive and fundamental role of splitting, or dissociation, in schizophrenia. All quotations from Bleuler (1950 [1911]) in this chapter are reproduced with permission of the International Universities Press.

I call dementia praecox "schizophrenia" because (as I hope to demonstrate) the "splitting" of the different psychic functions is one of its most important characteristics. For the sake of convenience, I use the word in the singular although it is apparent that the group includes several diseases. (p. 8)

Etiology of Schizophrenia

Bleuler was ambivalent about whether schizophrenia can arise as a response to the environment in the absence of a preexisting or underlying disease. He considered the underlying biomedical disease to be the true schizophrenia, and he believed that the disease was inherited. However, Bleuler (1950 [1911], p. 340) stated explicitly that the schizophrenia phenotype can occur in the absence of the phenotype: "Is there a schizophrenia without any hereditary *Anlage*? Probably."

At other points in his 1911 text, Bleuler stated that schizophrenia cannot be caused solely by psychological factors. Even when leaning toward that conclusion, however, Bleuler wrote at length about the fundamental role of the psychosocial environment, especially trauma, in the creation of symptoms, the course of the illness, and long-term prognosis. His views are consistent with the theory of a dissociative subtype of schizophrenia.

> We must add, however, that it is not absolutely necessary to assume the presence of a physical disease process. It is conceivable that the entire symptomatology may be psychically determined and that it may develop on the basis of slight quantitative deviations from the normal, just as in some people the disposition to hysterical symptoms is so strong that they become hysterical when confronted with the ordinary difficulties of life, whereas, in the average person, hysteria can develop only in consequence of a very severe psychic trauma. (Bleuler, 1950 [1911], pp. 461-462)

Although he exhibited some ambivalence in his views, Bleuler believed that schizophrenia is almost always based on an underlying biological disease. He thought that some cases could be induced by the environment in the absence of the underlying disease. Overall, however, he believed that the environment influences the phenomenology, prognosis, and treatment response of schizophrenia in a much more pervasive and fundamental manner than the "trigger" role it has in current versions of the diathesis-stress model.

The Role of Psychological Trauma

Bleuler repeatedly described the pervasive and fundamental role of psychological trauma in schizophrenia. He considered trauma to be a primary cause of the dissociation he observed in his patients, and he considered dissociation to be the fundamental phenomenon in schizophrenia.

According to Bleuler, the underlying disease process in schizophrenia is an inherited weakness of the psyche, an inability to maintain normal associations. In a patient with a high level of genetic loading, the core dissociation could arise with little or no environmental triggering. At the opposite end of the continuum, high levels of trauma are required to produce significant dissociation. This is a dose-response model with varying thresholds of endogenous dissociative susceptibility.

Bleuler believed that the greater the role of trauma in a case of schizophrenia, the better the prognosis. He never conducted any research involving statistical analysis, control or comparison groups, standardized psychometrics, or experimental designs. He was unable to demonstrate a relationship between trauma and psychosis because he was born a century too early and lacked the tools and measures available at the beginning of the twenty-first century.

Bleuler, as with all students of schizophrenia after him, was unable to demonstrate a diagnostically specific causal and underlying biological abnormality in his patients. He therefore considered, but in the end never accepted or rejected, the possibility that there is no underlying biomedical disease.

> Of course, even in the splitting off of affects, we are dealing with relative conditions. If the affects are strong, the dissociative tendencies need not be too pronounced in order to produce emotional devastation. Thus, in many cases of severe disease, we find that only quite ordinary everyday conflicts of life have caused marked deterioration; but in milder cases, the acute episodes may have been released by powerful affects. And quite

often, after a detailed analysis, we had to pose the question whether we are not merely dealing with the effect of a particularly powerful psychic trauma on a very sensitive person rather than with a disease in the narrow sense of the word. (Bleuler, 1950 [1911], p. 368)

Bleuler described the role of psychological trauma in case examples and vignettes. None of the vignettes rule out genetics and endogenous biology as contributing factors, but they do consistently evoke the theme of psychological trauma, which appears in many different cases throughout the text.

The contemporary literature on pathological dissociation emphasizes sexual abuse as a major form of trauma causing dissociative symptoms (Chu, 1998; Putnam, 1997). Bleuler described the role of sexual trauma in schizophrenia, although he placed less emphasis on it than we see in the dissociative disorders literature. This is to be expected, given the far lower level of attention to sexual abuse in 1911 than in contemporary Western cultures.

> . A patient hallucinated that her mother had complained about her to the patient's father; then the father "looked at her in a very strange way." He thrust a spear into her lower abdomen, at the same time dancing about in a very peculiar fashion. He was all black and completely nude. He often came to her in bed like that, all black, and occasionally he also appeared to her in the form of a bull. The patient related that her father had often beaten her—and wanted to abuse her sexually. He often played with her genitalia and must have gone even further. (Bleuler, 1950 [1911], p. 412)

The transparent meaning of the hallucinations in this case, combined with Bleuler's statement that there can be no hallucinations independent of their content (p. 349), points to the important role of sexual trauma in schizophrenia.

Descriptions of Thought Disorder

Bleuler described the dissociative subtype of schizophrenia explicitly and in great detail. He also provided descriptions of florid thought disorder. Such flagrant disorganization of language, unless it occurs on a transient basis, virtually rules out the dissociative subtype of schizophrenia.

The following sample from Bleuler's caseload is very unlike anything to be found in the journals of patients in treatment for DID:

> At Apell plain church-state, the people have customs and habits taken partly from glos-faith because the father wanted to enter new f. situation, since they believed the father had a Babeli comediation only with music. Therefore they went to the high Osetion and on the cabbage earth and all sorts of malice, and against everything good. On their inverted Osetion valley will come and within thus is the father righteousness. (Bleuler, 1950 [1911], p. 156)

The problem in Bleuler's typology is the absence of a dissociative subtype of schizophrenia. Patients such as the one just quoted clearly belong to a different subgroup. There is no possibility of doing psychotherapy with someone whose language is incoherent, scrambled, and idiosyncratic. However, other patients in the same overall diagnostic category of schizophrenia respond very well to verbal and behavioral interventions and to a positive, humane environment. This was true in Bleuler's time as it is today.

THE FUNDAMENTAL ROLE OF DISSOCIATION IN SCHIZOPHRENIA

In Bleuler, splitting and dissociation are synonyms. Dissociation can occur in schizophrenia due to an underlying disease process, as a reaction to the environment, or both. The symptoms of schizophrenia, including the four As, are secondary to the dissociation.

> The splitting is the fundamental prerequisite condition of most of the complicated phenomena of the disease. It is the splitting which gives the peculiar stamp to the entire symptomatology. However, behind this systematic splitting into defi-

nite idea-complexes, we have found a previous primary loosening of the associational structure which can lead to an irregular fragmentation of such solidly established elements as concrete ideas. The term, schizophrenia, refers to both kinds of splitting which often fuse in their effects. (Bleuler, 1950 [1911], p. 362)

What Gross understands by his term, "fragmentation (or disintegration) of consciousness" corresponds to what we call "splitting" . . . The term, "dissociation" has already been in use for a long time to designate similar observations and findings. (p. 363)

In several passages, Bleuler tries to differentiate between schizophrenia and hysteria. His criterion that splitting of concepts never occurs in "hysteria" is simply mistaken—it is present in every case of DID. Indeed, the disorder would be impossible without splitting of concepts, especially concepts of identity.

Writing in the same period, Janet (1965 [1907], 1977 [1901]) described the same patient population, called them hysterics, and concluded that dissociation was the fundamental phenomenon in hysteria. In the DSM-IV-TR, fragmented elements of Janet's hysteria are scattered throughout the manual, primarily appearing in somatization disorder, conversion disorder, histrionic personality disorder, and the dissociative disorders.

In my opinion, a large subgroup of the patients Bleuler diagnosed as suffering from schizophrenia are indistinguishable from Janet's hysterics, from the patients described in Breuer and Freud's (1986 [1895]) *Studies on Hysteria,* and from the patients I treat in my trauma programs (Ross, 1997). The "hysterical" elements of Bleuler's schizophrenia have been forgotten. They cannot be found in the contemporary literature on schizophrenia, except in case histories, where they are glossed over, not commented on, or ignored.

Contemporary accounts of Bleulerian splitting limit it to a split between thought and feeling or between reality and nonreality. In fact, splitting or dissociation affects all elements of psychic function in Bleuler's (1950 [1911]) schizophrenia, including the personality (Box 10.1).

**BOX 10.1. Psychological and physiological elements
that are dissociated in Bleuler's schizophrenia**

Attention	Will	Movement
Personality	Memory	Pain
Touch	Emotion	Arousal
Ideas	Voice	Personal name
Somatic sensations	Hallucinations	Physiological functions
(e.g., heart rate)

The possibility of splitting of attention is naturally a consequence of the personality split. (p. 371)

In a moderately stuporous patient, the pulse remained for some hours at one-hundred and forty, although usually it kept within normal limits. (p. 165)

Blockings and the influence of split-off complexes generally, often interfere with motility. (p. 448)

On the other hand, the lability of affect corresponds to his dissociated thinking. (pp. 44-45)

The autism is a direct consequence of the schizophrenic splitting of the psyche. (p. 373)

Because of the far-reaching split in the psychic functions, the affect becomes all-powerful in the realm of a certain complex of ideas; riticism and correction become impossible. Thus, within the split-off complexes, the affects create fantastic worlds for themselves ignoring reality, from which they select material suitable for their purposes. (p. 385)

The splitting of the personality is never more strikingly expressed than in the relation of the delusions to the remainder of the psyche. Part of that total complex which we call the ego, the "self," always remains alien to the delusions. This constellation accounts for the fact that the non-affected part of the ego may disbelieve and even criticize the delusions; on the other hand, the incorrigibility and senselessness of the delusions are precisely due to the fact that many associations contradictory to the delusional are simply not brought into any logical connection with it. (p. 127)

> The association-splitting can also lead to pathological ambivalences in which contradictory feelings or thoughts exist side by side without influencing each other. (p. 355)

Descriptions of dissociation such as those just quoted are not conclusive, however. It remains unclear whether Bleuler is describing full DSM-IV-TR DID. The following passages bring us closer to proof that Bleuler's (1950 [1911]) schizophrenia corresponds to DID.

> Not infrequently the delusions are split off from the personality in such a way that they appear to the patient as the product not of his own mental activity, but rather as the resultant workings of another psyche. (p. 128)

> The splitting of the psyche into several souls always leads to the greatest inconsistencies. (pp. 129-130)

> It is especially important to know that these patients carry on a kind of "double-entry bookkeeping" in many of their relationships. They know the real state of affairs as well as the falsified one and will answer according to the circumstances with one kind or the other type of orientation—or both together. (p. 56)

> [I]t is precisely the split-off part of the patient's personality which forces upon the other the hallucinations and their interpretation. (p. 310)

> Many thoughts are split off and absolutely incapable of establishing any associative contact with certain others. (p. 312)

Dissociative Identity Disorder Phenomena in Schizophrenia

If they were presented as quotations from a contemporary textbook of psychiatry, the following passages would lead 100 percent of readers to conclude that the patients being described have DID. These passages prove beyond a shadow of a doubt that Bleuler saw many cases of dissociative schizophrenia, and that these cases are indistinguishable from DSM-IV-TR DID.

> In every case we are confronted with a more or less clear-cut splitting of the psychic functions. If the disease is marked, the personality loses its unity; at different times different psychic complexes seem to represent the personality. Integration of different complexes and strivings appears insufficient or even lacking. The psychic complexes do not combine in a conglomeration of strivings with a unified resultant as they do in a healthy person; rather, one set of complexes dominates the personality for a time, while other groups or drives are "split off" and seem either partly or completely impotent. (p. 9)

> The delusion of being possessed is very commonly seen as a specific type of "double personality." (p. 123)

> Since any part of the ego may be split off and, on the other hand, since entirely alien concepts may be attached to it, the patients become "depersonalized." The person "loses his boundaries in time and space." The patients may identify themselves with some other person, even with inanimate objects, with a chair, with Switzerland. *Single emotionally charged ideas or drives attain a certain degree of autonomy so that the personality falls to pieces. These fragments can then exist side by side and alternately dominate the main part of the personality, the conscious part of the patient.* However, the patient may also become a definitely different person from a certain moment onwards. (p. 143, italics in original)

> Naturally such patients must speak of themselves in one of their two versions or they may speak in the third person of the other two. This sort of reference is here not merely an unusual or awkward figure of speech such as we may find in mental defectives or in children, but is the expression of a real alteration in personality. But even when such a splitting cannot be demonstrated, a patient may speak of himself only in the third person. Usually he designates himself by one of his several names. (p. 144)

Some of these patients are at any one time so consistently and so completely the one personality or the other, that they do not even think of the other person when they assume the part of one; the person whom they represent at the moment is considered as the natural one. (p. 144)

The patient, with whom one has just had a pleasant talk, suddenly becomes agitated, says what otherwise he does not believe, and distorts his logic entirely in terms of his anger. He is an entirely different person, only to return shortly to his former state. (p. 146)

In a few cases the "other" personality is marked by the use of different speech and voice. . . . Thus we have here two different personalities operating side by side, each one fully attentive. However, they are probably never completely separated from each other since one may communicate with both. (p. 147)

When the patients think of themselves as different persons, they utilize a correspondingly different tone of voice. One of our patients spoke with the voice of the child who wanted to emerge through the patient's mouth.

When specific "persons" speak through the patients, in various cases of automatic speech, each "person" has his own specific voice and distinct manner of speech. (p. 149)

Thus the patient appears to be split into as many different persons or personalities as they have complexes. (p. 361)

As the result of the splitting-off of independently operating complexes, the patient often feels as if another second self existed within himself. When the patient is ignorant of or instinctively rejects the pathological nature of such experiences, he is compelled to conclude that he is "possessed" or hypnotically influenced or some such thing. (p. 384)

The systematic splitting, with reference to personality, for example, may be found in many other psychotic conditions; in hysteria they are even more marked than in schizophrenia (multiple personalities). Definite splitting, however, in the sense that various personality fragments exist side by side in a state of clear orientation as to environment, will only be found in our disease. (pp. 298-299)

In the last passage there is an element of turf war. Bleuler is claiming that a large group of patients are his, have his disease, belong in his hospital, and require his diagnostic and treatment methods. To assert his claim to this territory, Bleuler tries to differentiate schizophrenia from hysteria, but he does so in an implausible, inconsistent, and self-contradictory fashion. The problem is that there is often no difference between DID and the dissociative subtype of schizophrenia—both are described in minute detail by Bleuler, and both were major elements of his caseload.

This is not simply a problem of unrecognized comorbidity, or of the need to reclassify some of Bleuler's patients as suffering from DID. The core phenomenology of the two disorders overlaps too often and too much for it to be simply a problem of comorbidity involving two discrete categories. That is why I propose a dissociative subtype of schizophrenia.

Given that 4 percent of general adult psychiatric inpatients have undiagnosed DID, while another 10 percent have undiagnosed, closely related forms of DDNOS, a question arises: how can the bulk of psychiatrists fail to notice DID, when it can often be diagnosed in less than an hour with a structured interview?

It might seem implausible that there are so many easily diagnosed but unrecognized cases of DID in the world's inpatient wards and outpatient clinics. It is not. Such cases were a major component of Bleuler's caseload. They are described explicitly and in minute detail —if psychiatrists can miss the obvious cases of DID in Bleuler, there is no reason we should expect them to diagnose cases correctly in the clinic. The myth that schizophrenia and split personality are separate and distinct has helped maintain a conversion agnosia for DID in psychiatry.

Bleuler's text was published nearly 100 years ago, and he has been regarded as a leading authority on schizophrenia ever since. To be blind to DID, however, it has simultaneously been necessary for psychiatrists to be blind to Bleuler. His phenomenology of schizophrenia has been forgotten because it refutes the proposition that DID is rare and distinct from schizophrenia.

The facts are as follows:

- Undiagnosed DID affects 4 percent of general adult psychiatric inpatients; many DID patients have received prior diagnoses of schizophrenia.
- Two-thirds of DID patients meet structured interview criteria for schizophrenia or schizoaffective disorder.
- One-quarter of schizophrenia patients meet structured interview criteria for DID.
- Bleuler described DID in minute and explicit detail.
- Bleuler's phenomenology of schizophrenia has been forgotten.

State Switching in Schizophrenia

In numerous case examples, Bleuler describes switches of state that are highly suggestive of undiagnosed DID. Even if full DID is not present in these cases, they provide florid examples of dissociative switches of state. They would therefore meet criteria for DDNOS, if not for full DID, on modern psychometric assessment. They would exhibit classical profiles of chronic, complex dissociation on the DES, DDIS, SCID-D, and MID.

> Stuporous patients can very suddenly become perfectly capable of playing chess correctly, or of writing and playing the piano rapidly, etc. A visit from the family may often induce such patients to "wake up" completely. (Bleuler, 1950 [1911]), p. 185)

> Thus a catatonic of long standing would show two alternating conditions during a single conversation with her. Her first condition was characterized by good orientation to her environment and a certain degree of insight; in her second state, she considered the doctor to be the devil, misinterpreted her environment in the same sense, and hid under the covers with tremendous anxiety. (p. 240)

> Special attention should be given to the frequently occurring sudden remissions in the very midst of an acute episode, partic-

ularly, in such as have the characteristics of marked delusional ideas or catatonia; such patients may then appear quite normal to a layman. (p. 249)

Amnesia in Schizophrenia

Dissociative amnesia is a major symptom of Bleuler's schizophrenia. The amnesia has psychological meaning and purpose, which is why it is likely dissociative and not organic. Of course, there is no definitive proof in these passages that the amnesia is dissociative rather than organic. Inversely, there is no evidence of a specific biological cause. The irrefutable point is, regardless of etiology, amnesia is a major phenomenon in Bleuler's schizophrenia.

The theory of a dissociative subtype of schizophrenia not only allows but predicts that some of the dissociative symptoms have an endogenous biological etiology; the validity of the subtype does not depend on theories of etiology, since it is defined phenomenologically, as are all other DSM-IV-TR diagnostic categories. As found in Bleuler (1950 [1911]), these quotes describe amnesia in his patients:

> The blocking of the recall of memories is a common occurrence during the examination of patients, and above all hinders the recall of those memories which are connected with emotionally accentuated complexes. (p. 60)

> After acute and agitated phases of the disease we frequently encounter an amnesia varying widely in intensity and extent. Sometimes the patients sense these lacunae and are then disposed to ascribe them to hypnosis or some other influence. (p. 140)

> A hebephrenic had two identical attacks with shaking and twisting of his limbs, turning of the eyeballs, facial pallor, foaming at the mouth. Each attack lasted several hours, and was followed by total amnesia. . . . A catatonic patient rolls her eyeballs, kicks with her feet, and foams at the mouth; duration: about two minutes, with total amnesia. (p. 178)

The dissociative amnesia in schizophrenia is intermingled with flashbacks, spontaneous abreactions, traumatic reenactments, age regressions, and other symptoms of PTSD. All of this phenomenology is seen daily in my trauma programs, where it is treated with behavioral and psychotherapeutic interventions.

These posttraumatic symptoms are core elements of Bleuler's phenomenology of schizophrenia and of his model of schizophrenia; they are not comorbidity because they are core aspects of schizophrenia. It is not a matter of the co-occurrence of discrete categories (environmental reaction versus endogenous biological disease), because the phenomenology used to define the two categories overlaps too much, and is too often the same thing.

Phenomena of Janet's Hysteria in Schizophrenia

Although Bleuler's entire text could be regarded as a treatise on Janet's hysteria, certain aspects of his phenomenology are particularly reminiscent of Janet, who is today regarded as the grandfather of the dissociative disorders field (Van der Hart and Friedman, 1989). In the following passages, somatoform and conversion symptoms are predominant. Bleuler's patients would have high scores on the Somatoform Dissociation Questionnaire (Nijenhuis, 1999). All of the quoted material quoted is from Bleuler (1950 [1911]).

> Even in well oriented patients one may often observe the presence of a complete *analgesia* which includes the deeper parts of the body as well as the skin. The patients intentionally or unintentionally incur quite serious injuries, pluck out an eye, sit down on a hot stove and receive severe gluteal burns, etc. . . . A hebephrenic student complained that often he could hear nothing of the lecture to which he was listening; he felt as if he had suddenly gone deaf. Another patient was suddenly unable to see, which he explained as the workings of some mysterious "influence." A catatonic woman felt "as if something struck her;" and suddenly it was as if her ears were plugged. She could hear sound only but could not make out any of the words. (p. 57)

> *Anorexia* is frequently accompanied in acute states by symptoms of "gastric catarrh" (coated tongue, foul breath, sometimes mild elevation of temperature). In chronic states, anorexia more often occurs without these accompanying symptoms. Alter-

nately with the anorexia (or by itself), we may observe *bulimia,* acutely or chronically. (p. 162)

Sleep is habitually disturbed. . . . Symptoms of *fatigue* are varied. (p. 169)

Headaches of long standing are very often found among the sensory disturbances which are part of the somatic symptoms. (p. 173)

Sometimes the symptoms have a clearly *hemiplegic character,* one half of the body slackening during the attack and seeming weaker afterwards . . . *fainting spells* . . . many of our patients were first sent to us with the diagnosis of epilepsy. . . . An older schizophrenic had her first epileptiform attack immediately after having observed, with great interest, a fit in an epileptic patient. (pp. 175-176)

Often enough, the entire automatic action is split off from the conscious personality of the patient. The limbs do something, the lips say something, of which the person is informed by his senses as if he were an observer during the action, as if he were a third person. In particular, writing and speaking often present themselves like this. Only these split-off actions are to be considered as automatisms in the full sense of the word. (p. 201)

The Ganser syndrome in schizophrenics is released by the same causes as in the hysterics. Prisoners being detained for judicial or medical examination are particularly afflicted with this syndrome. (p. 219)

Intercurrent episodes of agitation and excitement can also assume the form of fugues. Some patients may have been quite dependable in many respects, led a life devoid of desires and interests, yet suddenly they may run off, often getting quite far away. . . . Schizophrenic fugue (or wandering) states often give occasion for desertions from military units. (p. 226)

> There are many among them [hebephrenics] who, for years, were considered to be neurasthenics, or if women, hysterics. (p. 235)

> P. Janet speaks of *"abaissement du niveau mental"* in patients we would consider schizophrenic. (p. 380)

Except for the cases with florid thought disorders, there are no symptoms of schizophrenia in Bleuler that cannot be found in Janet's (1965 [1901], 1977 [1907]) books on hysteria, in Breuer and Freud's (1986 [1895]) *Studies on Hysteria,* or in the contemporary literature on DID (Ross, 1997). What Bleuler calls the mental state of schizophrenia, Janet calls the mental state of hystericals. What Bleuler calls the major symptoms of schizophrenia, Janet calls the major symptoms of hysteria.

In my opinion, catatonia is one of the most floridly "hysterical" symptoms in schizophrenia. The reason that the catatonic subtype of schizophrenia is far less common now than it was a century ago is that schizophrenic catatonia is more psychological than biological in origin. Catatonia probably spread within schizophrenia in much the way pseudoseizures spread at the Salpêtrière hospital in Paris while Charcot and Janet were there.

In contemporary DID, there is a low but consistent prevalence of pseudoseizures, but no florid catatonia. The cultural, psychological, and sociological reasons for the disappearance of catatonia would be a fascinating subject for a separate book.

Only Karen Gainer (1994), to my knowledge, among all mental health professionals who have read Bleuler since 1911, understood that Bleuler was describing DID. It was Gainer's presentation of her analysis at a conference paper session I chaired in 1992 that inspired me to read Bleuler. To my knowledge, Bleuler provides the richest description of the dissociative subtype of schizophrenia in the psychiatric literature—even the problem of accurate versus inaccurate memories (Ross, 1995, 1997) is well described.

The fact that people with schizophrenia often simultaneously meet criteria for DID has been forgotten since Bleuler, but on the other hand, it is still a well-understood fact. Kendler, Spitzer, and Williams (1990), in their reply to Rathbun and Rustagi (1990), state, "As they are undoubtedly aware, there are individuals with classic schizophrenia who claim to be 'inhabited' by other beings or personalities" (p. 375).

The basic clinical observation has not been forgotten, but there is no conceptual model for making sense of it in the contemporary schizophrenia literature. Rathbun and Rustagi (1990) argued that multiple personality disorder should be included in the differential diagnosis of schizophrenia and as an exclusion criterion in the DSM-IV diagnostic criteria.

Kendler, Spitzer, and Williams (1990) responded:

> A generic issue raised by the letter of Drs. Rathbun and Rustagi is the extent to which diagnostic criteria for relatively common disorders should be modified only to address the problems of differential diagnosis with respect to relatively rare disorders. Our own impression is that a textual acknowledgment that multiple personality disorder must be considered in the differential diagnosis of schizophrenialike states would be sufficient for DSM-IV and would be preferable to a modification of the schizophrenia criteria themselves. (p. 375)

Since DID affects about 1 percent of the general population and 4 percent of general adult psychiatric inpatients, and since about 3 percent of the general population belongs to the dissociative taxon (facts that were not available to Kendler, Spitzer, and Williams in 1990), it is now evident that the differential diagnosis of schizophrenia and DID is a major problem in psychiatry and for DSM-V. This has been true since Bleuler published his classic text in 1911, but until recently we have not had reliable measures of dissociation, a critical mass of literature, or a theoretical model to bring order, science, and testability to the problem.

Chapter 11

Positive Symptoms in Schizophrenia and Dissociative Identity Disorder

In this chapter, I present and discuss empirical data on the overlap between schizophrenia and DID; positive and negative symptoms in schizophrenia and DID; confusion between schizophrenia and DID among treating psychiatrists; cases of schizophrenia with and without childhood abuse; and psychotic symptoms in PTSD. I conclude by presenting data from a new sample of schizophrenic subjects that was analyzed to test the theory of a dissociative subtype of schizophrenia.

Positive symptoms of schizophrenia are more characteristic of DID than they are of schizophrenia. They may be more related to psychological trauma than they are to any endogenous biological disease process occurring in schizophrenia. The data in this chapter support the existence of a dissociative subtype of schizophrenia. They also disrupt and invalidate the two discrete categories described in Table 11.1.

DISTINCTION BETWEEN SCHIZOPHRENIA AND DID IN THE SCHIZOPHRENIA LITERATURE

The academic schizophrenia literature, as with information on the Internet, includes two supposedly distinct categories, schizophrenia and DID, as shown in Table 11.1. In fact, schizophrenia and DID are not distinct. They overlap a great deal. The reasons given in the schizophrenia literature for Bleuler's choice of the term *schizophrenia* are not based on his 1911 text—they have been told and retold as an urban legend version of Bleuler, with slight variations from teller to teller.

TABLE 11.1. Two distinct categories in the schizophrenia literature and on the Internet: schizophrenia and dissociative identity disorder

Schizophrenia	Dissociative identity disorder
No dissociation	Dissociation
Psychosis	No psychosis
Biological disease	Reaction to the psychosocial environment
Biological cause	Psychological cause
Genetic	Learned
Medication	Psychotherapy
1 percent of the population	Rare
Legitimate/mainstream	Questionable/fringe

It is understandable that support groups such as the National Alliance for the Mentally Ill (NAMI) and the Schizophrenia Society of Canada endorse the biomedical disease model of schizophrenia. Such groups include many members who are parents of schizophrenic children. There is probably an overrepresentation of parents of biological disease pathway schizophrenia, and a reciprocal underrepresentation of trauma pathway cases among members of such organizations.

Parents with schizophrenic children who have perpetrated chronic, severe neglect, family violence, and physical, sexual, and emotional abuse on their children are unlikely to be active in support groups. The endogenous biomedical disease model of schizophrenia probably fits many families of NAMI members fairly well. Such families, however, are probably a nonrandom and unrepresentative sample of all families with schizophrenic members. Academic psychiatry currently endorses an endogenous biomedical disease model of schizophrenia, to the virtually complete exclusion of the psychosocial environment. In my view, that is a scientific error; the biology of schizophrenia interacts with the enviroment much more than the unidirectional, endogenous model allows. I don't doubt that endogenous biomedical cases of schizophrenia exist, but I think they are a minority of the overall caseload.

Within the schizophrenia literature, the distinction between schizophrenia and DID is not a serious problem. The possibility of a relationship or overlap between the two disorders is not considered. For instance, Torrey et al. (1994) state, "The popular but incorrect image of schizophrenia as a 'split personality' also reflects a belief that schizophrenia changes the personality, even splitting it into parts" (p. 144).

Similarly, Pinals and Breier (1997) state,

> Although erroneously defined by laypeople as multiple personality disorder, this term means literally "splitting of the mind." Bleuler used the word to capture his belief that this mental illness was one in which different aspects of the psyche were split, which resulted in the classical symptoms he went on to describe. (p. 928)

Contemporary authorities on schizophrenia agree that schizophrenia is not multiple (DID) personality. However, they arrive at this agreement without reference to the relevant literature and without analysis or argument. Confusion between schizophrenia and split personality is regarded by authorities on schizophrenia as occurring only in the lay mind. The implication is that the distinction is clear and settled in the professional literature.

In fact the overlap between schizophrenia and multiple (DID) personality is an unrecognized but major problem in psychiatry. The overlap between the two disorders has been ignored in the schizophrenia literature because the pervasive and fundamental role of dissociation in Bleuler's schizophrenia has been forgotten, because DID has been regarded as rare, because dissociation has been relegated to the category of neurosis, and because schizophrenia has been defined as a biomedical brain disorder.

Neuroses, including hysteria, are reactions to the psychosocial environment, within the conceptual system of contemporary academic psychiatry, while schizophrenia is an endogenous biomedical disease with some degree of triggering by biological and physical factors in the environment.

To date, however, there is no specific genetic or biological criterion for schizophrenia. Not only is there no brain, blood, chromosomal, or metabolic abnormality that is specific for the disorder, there is no biological marker that even approaches minimal sensitivity and specificity to be used as an aid to clinical diagnosis. There is no lab test for schizophrenia, and no conclusive scientific evidence that it is an endogenous biomedical disorder. Data on concordance in monozygotic twins prove conclusively that schizophrenia is primarily an environmentally induced disorder.

Despite these scientific facts, the endogenous biomedical causation of schizophrenia is regarded as proven within psychiatry. The public has been taught accordingly by psychiatrists. Given the assumptions of their conceptual system, contemporary authorities agree that schizophrenia cannot be caused by events within a child's family. In two books on the causes of schizophrenia, therefore, childhood sexual abuse is not mentioned once (Gottesman, 1991; Torrey et al., 1994). Childhood trauma is not relevant to the etiology, course, treatment, or prognosis of schizophrenia in the contemporary schizophrenia literature.

The clear differentiation of schizophrenia from MPD is endorsed on many Web sites and sources of public information. For instance, at <www.mentalhealth.com>, under a heading "SCHIZOPHRENIA IS," the visitor is informed that schizophrenia is "a brain disease, with concrete and specific symptoms due to physical and biochemical changes in the brain," and is "almost always treatable with medication." Under the heading "SCHIZOPHRENIA IS _NOT_," the visitor is advised that the illness is not "split personality," and is not "caused by childhood trauma, bad parenting, or poverty."

At <www.schizophrenia.com>, the visitor is advised, "Schizophrenia is not a split personality, a rare and very different disorder. Like cancer and diabetes, schizophrenia has a biological basis; it is not caused by bad parenting or personal weakness."

Similarly, <http://.faculty.washington.edu./chudler/schiz>, states,

> People who are schizophrenic do **NOT** have multiple personalities. In 1911, Eugen Bleuler, first used the word "schizophrenia." Although the word schizophrenia does come from the Greek words meaning "split" and "mind," schizophrenics do not have split personalities. This misunderstanding has caused many people to misuse the term schizophrenia. The "split mind"

refers to the way that schizophrenics are split off from reality; schizophrenics cannot tell what is real and what is not.

At <www.mentalhealth.com>, in a joint publication of Health Canada and the Schizophrenia Society of Canada, titled *Schizophrenia: A Handbook for Families,* the reader is informed,

> The term "schizophrenia" was introduced in 1911 by a Swiss psychiatrist, Eugen Bleuler. The word comes from the Greek schizo meaning "split" and phrenia meaning "mind." Bleuler wanted to convey the split between what is perceived, what is believed, and what is objectively real. He did not mean that the person with schizophrenia is split into two personalities, but that there is a splitting away of the personality from reality. The concept of "split," however, has led to schizophrenia being confused with multiple personality, a less common and very different disorder, much publicized through such stories as *Dr. Jekyll and Mr. Hyde, The Three Faces of Eve,* and *Sybil.*

The NAMI Web site, <www.nami.org>, endorses the same view in its booklet, "Understanding Schizophrenia": "Like cancer or diabetes, schizophrenia is a complex, chronic medical illness affecting different people in different ways. Schizophrenia is not caused by bad parenting or personal weakness. A person with schizophrenia does *not* have a 'split personality.' "

The Schizophrenia Society of Canada states on its Web site, <www.schizophrenia.ca>, that schizophrenia "is a *treatable* biochemical brain disease" and that "it is NOT: The fault of the person or their family." In a bulletin posted on the Schizophrenia Society of Canada Web site titled, "Recognizing Schizophrenia for What It Really Is," the following statement is made: "Schizophrenia is not a mental health issue. Mental health issues involve people who are disturbed by life. Schizophrenia is a biological disease of the brain." Elsewhere in the bulletin, it states that "the illness should be thought of as a disease in the same sense as cancer and heart disease."

A substantial body of data refutes the endogenous biomedical disease model of schizophrenia and the existence of the two dichotomized categories shown in Table 11.1. The same data support the existence of a dissociative subtype of schizophrenia characterized by high levels of psychological trauma. I now review that body of research data. Decades of neglect, violence, and physical, sexual, emotional, and verbal abuse can markedly increase the risk for dissociative schizophrenia—within my theory, I classify such behavior as "bad parenting"

DATA ON THE OVERLAP
BETWEEN SCHIZOPHRENIA AND DID

The two supposedly distinct categories shown in Table 11.1, schizophrenia and DID, in fact share many symptoms and characteristics. Evidence comes from a variety of sources, one of which is the prior diagnoses of schizophrenia given to patients in treatment for DID (see Table 11.2). Whichever is the accurate and whichever the inaccurate diagnosis, there is confusion and overlap between the two categories at the level of clinical diagnosis and treatment.

Putnam et al. (1986) reported a series of 100 patients with MPD, of whom just under 50 percent had received a prior diagnosis of schizophrenia from a psychiatrist. In my own series (Ross, Norton, and Wozney, 1989) of 236 cases, 40.8 percent had a prior diagnosis of schizophrenia. The patients in my series with a prior diagnosis of schizophrenia also had higher rates of suicide attempts; overdoses; self-inflicted injuries; wrist slashing; inpatient treatment; and treatment with antipsychotic medications, antidepressants, nonbenzodiazepine sedatives, benzodiazepines, lithium, and electroconvulsive therapy (Ross and Norton, 1988), as shown in Table 11.3. They had been in the mental

TABLE 11.2. Frequency of a previous diagnosis of schizophrenia and treatment with antipsychotic medications and ECT in two series of MPD cases (in percent)

Previous diagnosis and treatment	Series 1 (N = 236)	Series 2 (N = 102)
Diagnosis of schizophrenia	40.8	26.5
Treatment with neuroleptics	54.5	57.0
Treatment with ECT	12.1	16.7

ECT = electroconvulsive therapy

TABLE 11.3. Previous treatment of multiple personality disorder patients with a past diagnosis of schizophrenia

Treatment	Past diagnosis (N = 81) (%)	No past diagnosis (N = 96) (%)	p
Psychotherapy	89.7	88.5	NS
Inpatient	88.8	68.8	.002
Neuroleptic	88.5	36.5	.00001
Antidepressant	87.2	62.1	.0001
Nonbenzodiazepine sedative	75.0	52.6	.008
Benzodiazepine	58.8	56.4	NS
Lithium	36.2	12.8	.00001
Electroconvulsive therapy	20.3	7.5	.05

Source: Ross and Norton, 1988, Table 2, p. 41. Reproduced by permission of Dissociative Disorders Research Publications Limited.

health system longer prior to diagnosis and had received more previous diagnoses: affective disorder (77.1 percent); personality disorder (71.8 percent); anxiety disorder (51.5 percent); and substance abuse (45.2 percent) were the most common comorbid diagnoses.

My series of 236 cases was based on a questionnaire mailed out to all members of the Canadian Psychiatric Association and the ISSD. The respondents were a mixture of specialists in dissociative disorders and general psychiatrists. Although the ISSD members had seen most cases, the phenomenology of multiple personality was remarkably consistent when I compared cases reported by Canadian generalists to those reported by American specialists (Ross, Norton, and Fraser, 1989).

In the two large series of multiple personality cases (Putnam et al., 1986; Ross, Norton, and Wozney, 1989), previous diagnoses of schizophrenia and prior treatment with antipsychotic medications and electroconvulsive therapy (ECT) demonstrate that prior treating clinicians assessed these individuals as suffering from severe mental illnesses with psychotic symptoms. This in turn proves, within the limitations of the data, that the two supposedly distinct categories shown in Table 11.1 are in fact highly confused and overlapping in clinical practice.

As mentioned, I subdivided my series of 236 cases into two categories (Ross and Norton, 1988): those with (N = 81) and without (N = 96) a prior diagnosis of schizophrenia. The remaining 59 individuals in the series of 236 did not specify whether they did or did not have a prior diagnosis of schizophrenia, or were uncertain. A prior diagnosis of schizophrenia meant a more complex treatment history. This suggests that the 81 individuals who had received diagnoses of both MPD and schizophrenia represented a severe variant of schizophrenia.

My argument is that three conclusions are consistent with the existing data:

1. DID is a common true positive diagnosis among people in treatment for a false positive diagnosis of schizophrenia.
2. The two conditions commonly co-occur.
3. There is a dissociative subtype of schizophrenia, and an independent diagnosis of DID is not necessary.

I learned from my mail-out survey of treating clinicians (Ross and Norton, 1988) that MPD patients with prior diagnoses of schizophrenia are more complicated, disturbed, and difficult to treat than those without that prior diagnosis. Also, within the methodological limitations of such a survey, I learned what I already knew clinically: the same individuals often receive a diagnosis of schizophrenia from one clinician but a diagnosis of MPD from another.

Since the pool of clinicians willing to make a diagnosis of MPD was far smaller than the number willing to make a diagnosis of schizophrenia in the 1980s, I concluded that there was probably a large number of people in the mental health system with false positive diagnoses of schizophrenia and false negative diagnoses of multiple personality disorder. Many of these people, I suspected, could participate in sustained, intensive psychotherapy designed to treat their psychotic symptoms, including their auditory hallucinations.

I decided to investigate these suspicions with a series of research studies. The first task was to develop a reliable structured interview for the dissociative disorders, which resulted in the DDIS (Ross,

1989, 1997). Using the DDIS, I conducted a series of studies in which I compared MPD patients to other diagnostic groups and investigated the frequency of undiagnosed dissociative disorders in various clinical groups and the general population (Ross, 1997).

My aim was, in part, to study both the similarities and the differences between schizophrenia and MPD, which was renamed DID in the DSM-IV (American Psychiatric Association, 1994). I wanted to know which measures and symptom clusters were common to the two disorders, and which were more characteristic of one or the other. I also wanted to study the rates of reported childhood physical and sexual abuse among patients with the two disorders.

The data presented in this chapter are not conclusive. They require replication, refinement, and validation with other measures and methodologies. However, they are of sufficient rigor and mass to prove that the dissociative subtype of schizophrenia is a theory worthy of serious investigation. There is no need for critics to point out that it is not supported by sufficient data—the purpose of the theory is to stimulate research on its epidemiology, phenomenology, biology, and treatment.

In Tables 11.4, 11.5, and 11.6, I compare 166 patients with MPD (Ross et al., 1992) to 83 patients with long-standing, stable clinical diagnoses of schizophrenia (Ross, Anderson, and Clark, 1994). The three categories of abuse reported in Table 11.4 are sexual abuse, physical abuse, and physical and/or sexual abuse. Thus the rates of physical and sexual abuse are available separately and combined. It is clear from Table 11.4 that MPD patients report far higher rates of

TABLE 11.4. A comparison of schizophrenia and multiple personality disorder (MPD) on the Dissociative Disorders Interview Schedule: childhood trauma histories

Item	MPD (N = 166) % positive	Schizophrenia (N = 83) % positive	Chi-square	p
Physical abuse	78.3	31.1	81.831	.00001
Sexual abuse	84.3	25.3	50.221	.00001
Physical and/or sexual abuse	91.0	44.6	61.884	.0001

TABLE 11.5. A comparison of schizophrenia and multiple personality disorder (MPD) on the Dissociative Disorders Interview Schedule: Axis I and II diagnoses

Item	MPD (N = 166) % positive	Schizophrenia (N = 83) % positive	Chi-square	p
Psychogenic amnesia	75.9	36.1	35.701	.00001
Psychogenic fugue	13.9	3.6	5.159	.03
Depersonalization disorder	60.8	28.9	21.304	.00001
MPD	94.6	25.3	126.906	.00001
Somatization disorder	39.8	4.8	31.719	.00001
Substance abuse	51.2	43.4	1.063	NS
Depression	89.8	53.0	40.781	.00001
Borderline personality disorder	61.4	21.7	33.459	.00001

childhood physical and sexual abuse than those with schizophrenia. However, the base rate for physical and/or sexual abuse in the general population on the DDIS is 12.6 percent (Ross, 1991). Schizophrenia is linked to childhood trauma, but the association is not as strong as it is for MPD. Based on trauma histories, multiple personality could be a severe variant of schizophrenia, rather than a separate entity.

Different conclusions could be drawn from Table 11.5, depending on one's point of view. If we assume that the clinical diagnoses of MPD are all valid, then the sensitivity of the DDIS is 94.6 percent, which is excellent. What about the 25.3 percent of patients in treatment for schizophrenia who met DDIS and DSM-III-R criteria for MPD? Are these true or false positive diagnoses? It is impossible to tell from the methodology of the study because I did not conduct independent clinical interviews of the schizophrenic subjects.

In research conducted to date, 25 to 40 percent of subjects in treatment for schizophrenia report chronic, complex dissociation and meet DSM-IV-TR criteria for complex dissociative disorders. Future research must include clinical interviews, because the existing DSM-IV-TR categories, structured interviews and symptom measures cannot sort DID and schizophrenia patients into two discrete categories.

TABLE 11.6. A comparison of schizophrenia and multiple personality disorder (MPD) on the Dissociative Disorders Interview Schedule: symptom clusters

Symptom cluster	MPD (N = 166) average score or number of symptoms	Schizophrenia (N = 83) average score or number of symptoms	*t*	*p*
DES score	39.7	14.2	10.929	.00001
Somatic	14.1	2.8	12.846	.00001
Schneiderian	6.5	4.6	4.451	.00001
Secondary features of MPD	10.2	3.6	14.351	.00001
Borderline criteria	5.1	2.6	8.077	.00001
ESP/paranormal experiences	5.3	4.5	1.736	NS

Note: DES = Dissociative Experiences Scale

As for the trauma histories, the Axis I and II comorbidity profiles of schizophrenia are less severe than those of MPD, but the rates of comorbidity in schizophrenia are far higher than the base rates in the general population. Again, MPD looks like a severe variant of schizophrenia. The confusion and overlap between the two disorders is not dispelled when structured interviews are used or when DSM diagnostic criteria are applied—in fact, such procedures confirm the confusion and overlap.

It is interesting that substance abuse is the only comorbid diagnosis as common in schizophrenia as in MPD. Although no scientific conclusion can be drawn from this finding, my personal belief is that drugs and alcohol help the subjects cope with the misery of their lives, which overall is about equal in schizophrenia and MPD.

The symptom clusters in the DDIS follow the same pattern as the trauma histories and Axis I and II comorbidity. My prediction is that future research will confirm this pattern with a variety of measures and methodology—DID behaves as a severe variant of schizophrenia on all measures, with considerable overlap between the two groups. Positive symptoms of schizophrenia (Schneiderian symptoms) occur in both disorders but are more characteristic of DID than of schizo-

phrenia. The data do not support the existence of two discrete categories, according to my analysis.

As with substance abuse, one cannot reach a scientific conclusion
as to why ESP/paranormal experiences are equally common in the
two disorders. I suspect that this set of subjective experiences may be
equally characteristic of the endogenous biological and exogenous
trauma pathways to psychosis. Why this should be, I don't know.

SCID-D Data on Dissociative Symptoms and Diagnoses in Schizophrenia

The other structured interview for diagnosing dissociative disorders is the SCID-D Steinberg, 1995; Steinberg, Rounsaville, and
Cicchetti, 1990). The SCID-D, similar to the DES and DDIS, has sufficient reliability and validity to appear in the American Psychiatric
Association's *Handbook of Psychiatric Measures* (Pincus et al.,
2000). Steinberg et al. (1994) administered the SCID-D to nineteen
individuals with DID and twenty-eight with stable clinical diagnoses
of schizophrenia. Their intention was to demonstrate that the SCID-
D can differentiate the two disorders, and that DID patients have
more dissociative symptoms.

Steinberg et al. (1994) were successful in demonstrating these two
facts. However, for my purposes, the opposite finding is of more interest. It is true that the SCID-D can differentiate DID from schizophrenia, and that DID subjects score higher on all the subscales of the
SCID-D. However, individuals with schizophrenia score far above
general population norms on all subscales of the SCID-D.

The data from Steinberg et al. (1994), shown in Table 11.7, suggest
that something on the order of 32.1 percent of schizophrenics experience moderate or severe identity alteration, a figure close to the 25.3
percent who meet DDIS criteria for MPD.

Haugen and Castillo (1999) administered the SCID-D to fifty psychotic outpatients at a community mental health center in Hawaii,
thirty-five with schizophrenia, and fifteen with schizoaffective disorder. The fifty subjects included twenty-seven Asian Americans, nineteen Pacific Islanders, and four European Americans. Their findings
are shown in Table 11.8.

Haugen and Castillo's (1999) sample is racially and geographi-
cally distinct from most studies done in the mainland United States,
which involve mostly Caucasian subjects. Twenty-eight percent of

TABLE 11.7. A comparison of schizophrenia and dissociative identity disorder (DID) on the Structured Clinical Interview for DSM-IV Dissociative Disorders (SCID-D)

	% with moderate to severe symptoms	
Symptom scale	DID (N = 19)	Schizophrenia (N = 28)
Amnesia	94.7	57.1
Depersonalization	100.0	57.1
Derealization	100.0	42.9
Identity confusion	100.0	46.4
Identity alteration	100.0	32.1
SCID-D total score	100.0	28.6

Source: Adapted from Steinberg et al., 1994.

TABLE 11.8. Structured Clinical Interview for DSM-IV Dissociative Disorders (SCID-D) data on 50 patients with clinical diagnoses of schizophrenia (N = 35) or schizoaffective disorder (N = 15)

Dissociative disorder	Number positive for diagnosis	SCID-D total scores
Dissociative amnesia	2 (4%)	8.00
Depersonalization disorder	4 (8%)	9.50
DDNOS	7 (14%)	12.43
Dissociative trance disorder	11 (22%)	15.73
DID	7 (14%)	18.71
No dissociative disorder	19 (38%)	6.05

Note: DDNOS = dissociative disorder not otherwise specified; DID = dissociative identity disorder

the subjects met criteria for DID or DDNOS on the SCID-D, which is very consistent with the DDIS data in Table 11.5 and the SCID-D data in Table 11.7. As well, the SCID-D total score differentiated the various subtypes of dissociative disorder, as it was designed to do by Steinberg (1994), even though all subjects had schizophrenia or schizoaffective disorder. This finding adds additional validity to the conclusion that subjects with schizophrenia are often in the dissociative taxon, which in turn supports the validity of the dissociative subtype of schizophrenia.

Data indicate that the positive symptoms of schizophrenia are more characteristic of DID than of schizophrenia. This is a consistent and well-replicated finding in the dissociative disorders literature. It is a major problem because these symptoms are not included in the diagnostic criteria for DID but are the only symptoms required by the DSM-IV-TR to make a diagnosis of schizophrenia. The DSM-IV-TR states that if voices keep up a running commentary on the person's thoughts or behavior, or comment on each other, then no other symptom is required to make the diagnosis.

The fact that positive symptoms of schizophrenia are more characteristic of DID is not a problem within the schizophrenia field because of the myth that DID is rare and clearly differentiated from schizophrenia. Once this myth is dispelled, the need for a major revision of the DSM criteria for both schizophrenia and DID follows logically.

Data on Positive and Negative Symptoms in Schizophrenia and DID

The available data demonstrate that positive symptoms are more common in DID than in schizophrenia. The picture concerning negative symptoms is less clear because results in studies to date are not consistent. In each direction, the difference is a matter of degree rather than of discrete categories. In order to create empirically based, truly discrete categories, one might define the dissociative subtype of schizophrenia as a score above a certain cutoff on positive symptoms and below a cutoff on negative symptoms. Inversely, the nondissociative subtype could consist of individuals scoring below a cutoff on positive symptoms and above a cutoff on negative symptoms. Alternatively, scores on the DES could define dissociative and nondissociative subtypes of schizophrenia.

Receiver operating curves could be constructed for different measures and samples, and they could then generate diagnostic criteria, or, alternatively, weighted item scores could be used. A receiver operating curve plots the trade-offs between sensitivity and specificity at various cutoff scores on a measure. For instance, a DES cutoff score of 20 might detect 80 percent of the DID subjects in a sample, but would also incorrectly identify a large number of people as having DID. A cutoff score of 30 would miss more cases of DID but would yield fewer false positives. These approaches have been applied to the DES (Carlson et al., 1993; Waller, Putnam, and Carlson, 1996; Waller and Ross, 1997). Whatever the mathematical methodology, the research criteria would have to generate diagnostic criteria that were clear and simple enough to be used in the clinic.

The MID (Dell, 2002) is a computer-scored inventory with excellent reliability and validity. It generates a set of subscales and validity scales that can be displayed on a graph in a format similar to an MMPI profile. Laddis et al. (2001) used the MID in a study of thirty-five subjects with DID and twenty subjects with schizophrenia who were not currently actively psychotic. They asked the schizophrenic subjects to respond twice to each question, once for their current mental state, and once for their mental state during their last episode of active psychosis. Their findings are shown in Table 11.9.

A "made impulse" is experienced as coming from another person, power, or force outside the self. The person feels "made" to feel a feeling, act on an impulse, or think a thought.

All scores for DID versus schizophrenia in remission were significant at $p < .05$. For DID versus active psychosis, voices commenting,

TABLE 11.9. A comparison of schizophrenia and dissociative identity disorder (DID) on the Multidimensional Inventory of Dissociation (MID) (average MID scale scores)

Symptom	DID (N = 35)	Schizophrenia active (N = 20)	Schizophrenia in remission (N = 20)
Voices arguing	71.5	48.5	27.0
Voices commenting	61.4	26.6	21.4
Made feelings	69.2	34.5	22.1
Made impulses	66.2	34.4	24.3
Made actions	61.1	33.2	21.8
Influences on the body	48.8	20.5	16.3
Thought withdrawal	56.2	30.1	20.4
Thought insertion	59.5	35.8	22.5

made feelings, made impulses, and influences on the body were different at $p < .05$. Thus, the only required DSM-IV-TR positive symptom criterion for schizophrenia, voices commenting, is more characteristic of DID than of even the active psychotic phase of schizophrenia, according to the MID.

As for all the other data in this chapter, the MID data require replication and further study of their concurrent validity with other measures. However, the odds that significantly different findings will emerge from such studies are, in my view, minimal. More work is needed to prove the validity and generalizability of the initial findings, but the pattern is clear from the existing data reviewed in this chapter.

Kurt Schneider's (1959) eleven first-rank symptoms of schizophrenia were said by him to be pathognomonic of schizophrenia. Although this absolute specificity of first-rank symptoms has been abandoned, the DSM-IV-TR still regards voices commenting as so characteristic of schizophrenia that it is the only symptom required to make the diagnosis. The available data indicate that this symptom in fact has superior sensitivity and specificity as a diagnostic criterion for DID.

The PANSS (Kay, Opler, and Fiszbein, 1994; Pincus et al., 2000) was developed to measure the positive and negative symptoms of schizophrenia. Similar to the MID, it demonstrates that the positive symptoms of schizophrenia are more characteristic of DID than of schizophrenia. In addition, it demonstrates that negative symptoms are more characteristic of schizophrenia than of DID. This is an important finding for clinical and conceptual reasons, but also because it rules out an indiscriminate positive response bias by DID subjects.

Ellason and Ross (1995) administered the PANSS to 108 subjects with DID and compared the scores to norms for schizophrenia from the PANSS manual (Kay, Opler, and Fiszbein, 1994), as shown in Table 11.10. The composite score on the PANSS is the sum of the positive and negative symptom scores. The general scale measures a broad range of symptomatology—scores on this scale should be higher in the dissociative subtype of schizophrenia, as they should be for other measures of general psychopathology.

In order to investigate further the frequency of Schneiderian symptoms in MPD and schizophrenia, I conducted a review of the literature (Ross, Miller, Bjornson, et al., 1990). I found twelve series of schizophrenics and three series of MPD patients in which the prevalence and/or frequency of Schneiderian symptoms was reported (see Table 11.11). The average number of Schneiderian symptoms is higher in MPD than in schizophrenia, and so is the prevalence of having one or more symptoms. Indeed, the most remarkable finding of the literature review was that only 55.5 percent of 2,576 schizophrenic subjects in twelve series reported any Schneiderian symptoms.

TABLE 11.10. Comparison of schizophrenia and dissociative identity disorder (DID) on the Positive and Negative Syndrome Scale

Syndrome scale	DID (N = 108) average score	Schizophrenia (N = 240) average score	*t*	*p*
Positive	23.8	19.9	5.80	.00001
Negative	17.1	21.8	7.19	.00001
Composite	7.2	−1.9	10.36	.00001
General	50.1	39.7	10.02	.00001

Source: Ellason, J. W., and Ross, C. A. (1995). Positive and negative symptoms in dissociative identity disorder and schizophrenia. *Journal of Nervous and Mental Disease*, 183(4): 236-241. Table 3 reprinted by permission of Lippincott Williams & Wilkins.

TABLE 11.11. Prevalence and frequency of Schneiderian symptoms in schizophrenia and multiple personality disorder (MPD) in large case series

	MPD	Schizophrenia
	(N = 368)	(N = 1,739)
Average number of symptoms	4.9	1.3
	(N = 368)	(N = 2,576)
Subjects with one or more symptoms	87.0%	55.5%

Source: Adapted from Ross, Miller, Bjornson, et al., 1990.

I also tabulated the number of subjects having up to a possible total of eleven Schneiderian symptoms in three series of schizophrenics and one series of 102 cases of MPD. I found that many more schizophrenics than MPD patients had zero to four symptoms. Also, many MPD patients had nine or more symptoms, which was rare in schizophrenia.

According to the available data, the more symptoms of schizophrenia patients have, the less likely it is that they have schizophrenia, and the more likely it is that they have MPD. In fact, in some case series only one-third of the schizophrenic subjects had any Schneiderian symptoms at all.

If they were taken seriously, these findings would necessitate a revision of the DSM-IV-TR criteria for schizophrenia. In the DSM-IV-TR, schizophrenia can be diagnosed solely on the basis of symptoms that are more characteristic of DID (the A criteria). All the other DSM-IV-TR criteria for schizophrenia are either exclusion criteria or diagnostically nonspecific (duration of six months and a requirement for occupational or social deterioration, which can happen in countless diseases).

A regression analysis in a general population sample (Ross and Joshi, 1992) interviewed with the DDIS found that a history of physical and/or sexual abuse was a powerful predictor of the number of Schneiderian symptoms reported (beta weight = 0.51). Subjects in the general population with no Schneiderian symptoms reported an 8.1 percent rate of childhood physical and/or sexual abuse, compared to 45.7 percent in those reporting three or more symptoms. The relationship between trauma and symptoms of schizophrenia holds in a variety of clinical samples and in the general population in studies conducted to date, with no published exceptions to this pattern.

Data on the Differences Between Cases of Schizophrenia with and Without Childhood Abuse

Another way to look at the problem is to divide cases of schizophrenia into those reporting childhood abuse and those not reporting it. The differences between the abused and nonabused schizophrenic groups are shown in Tables 11.12 and 11.13 (Ross, Anderson, and Clark, 1994).

TABLE 11.12. A comparison of schizophrenia patients with and without reported childhood abuse on the Dissociative Experiences Scale (DES), Dissociative Disorders Interview Schedule (DDIS), and Positive and Negative Syndrome Scale (PANSS)

Measure	Abuse* (N = 37)	No abuse* (N = 46)	t	p
DES	21.6	8.5	4.8	.001
DDIS				
Schneiderian	6.3	3.3	3.9	.001
Somatic	4.7	1.3	3.9	.001
Secondary features of MPD	5.3	2.3	4.9	.001
Borderline	4.1	1.5	5.8	.001
ESP/paranormal	6.6	2.8	5.0	.001
Amnesia	2.5	1.2	5.7	.001
PANSS				
Positive	20.4	15.7	3.2	.002
Negative	−17.7	−21.0	1.9	.06
Composite	2.6	−5.3	4.0	.001

* Average score

Source: Adapted from Ross, Anderson, and Clark, 1994.

Note: MPD = multiple personality disorder

In this study, all subjects had stable, long-term diagnoses of schizophrenia and were in treatment at a university teaching hospital in Winnipeg, Canada, or at a provincial mental hospital in Selkirk, Canada. They were interviewed with the DES, DDIS, and PANSS. The same pattern was observed as in other studies. The schizophrenic subjects reporting child abuse had more dissociative, somatic, borderline, and ESP/paranormal symptoms. They also had more Schneiderian symptoms on the DDIS, and higher positive symptom scores and lower negative symptom scores on the PANSS. Thus, positive symptoms seemed to be caused as much by trauma as by any presumed endogenous disease process.

Based on this body of data, I conclude that there are at least two pathways to positive symptoms of psychosis: an endogenous disease pathway and a trauma pathway. The trauma pathway seems to predominate in both DID and schizophrenia. The negative symptoms of

TABLE 11.13. A comparison of schizophrenia patients with and without reported childhood abuse on the Diagnostic Interview Schedule (DIS)

DIS symptom	Abuse (%) (N = 37)	No abuse (%) (N = 46)	Chi-square	p
Ideas of reference	77.1	39.1	10.1	.002
Voices commenting	68.6	26.1	12.9	.001
Paranoid ideation	54.3	26.1	5.5	.02
Thought insertion	48.6	17.4	7.7	.006
Visual hallucinations	45.7	21.7	4.2	.04
Reading someone else's mind	37.1	13.0	5.2	.03

schizophrenia are more likely to be endogenous in origin than the positive symptoms.

Table 11.13 shows that this pattern is not an artifact of the DDIS or the PANSS because it is found when the Diagnostic Interview Schedule (DIS) is administered (Ross, Anderson, and Clark, 1994). I predict that this pattern of higher rates of positive symptoms in severely traumatized schizophrenics will hold for all measures of psychotic symptoms available in the literature.

Spitzer, Haug, and Freyberger (1997) studied the rates of dissociative symptoms in German schizophrenic patients with predominantly positive symptoms (N = 15) and predominantly negative symptoms (N = 12) on the PANSS. The average DES score was 21.1 for the positive symptom group and 9.2 for the negative group ($p < .002$). The correlation between scores on the DES and on the hallucinatory behavior scale of the PANSS was 0.60 among the twenty-seven patients. On the SCL-90, the average psychoticism score for the positive symptom group was 1.55, while for the negative symptom group it was 0.74 ($p < .02$).

Although more replications are required in a variety of samples with a range of different measures, a critical mass of data is available in the literature. The findings to date are consistent. Trauma, dissociation, and positive symptoms of schizophrenia are common both in people with DID and in people with schizophrenia. Positive symptoms of schizophrenia are more characteristic of DID. There is no definitive scientific proof for any causal pathway for positive symptoms in schizophrenia, but the evidence supporting a trauma pathway is at least as strong as that for any other proposed etiological pathway.

Data on Psychosis and Post-Traumatic Stress Disorder

Shaner and Eth (1989) and Lundy (1992) described cases in which PTSD seemed to occur in reaction to the trauma of psychosis. Earlier reports by Jeffries (1977), Domash and Sparr (1982), Waldfogel and Mueser (1988), and Mueser and Butler (1987) had already explored the relationship between psychosis and PTSD, as did a subsequent article by Williams-Keeler, Milliken, and Jones (1994).

Mueser and Butler found that a higher proportion of Hispanic Vietnam veterans with PTSD (60 percent) reported auditory hallucinations than did non-Hispanic veterans with PTSD (10 percent). Overall, veterans with auditory hallucinations had higher combat exposure scores than those without. They also found that veterans without auditory hallucinations responded better to flooding used as a therapeutic exposure technique. Their findings highlight the complex interaction of trauma dosage, cultural variables, psychotic symptoms, and treatment response.

Butler et al. (1996) studied twenty Vietnam veterans with PTSD and eighteen Vietnam veterans without PTSD. The veterans with PTSD had much higher scores on the SCL-90, indicating greater symptoms across a wide range. They scored higher on three scales of the SAPS, hallucinations, delusions, and bizarre behavior, but lower on the fourth scale, formal thought disorder. The only scale of the SANS on which the PTSD group scored higher was avolition/apathy. Wilcox, Briones, and Suess (1991) likewise found that Vietnam veterans with PTSD who also reported auditory hallucinations were more likely to be Hispanic (chi-square = 49.92; $p < .001$).

A small number of studies have consistently found high rates of PTSD among psychotic subjects. Shaw, McFarlane, and Bookless (1997) found postpsychotic PTSD in 52 percent of forty-five subjects recovering from hospitalization for a psychotic episode.

In a later study of forty-two people hospitalized for psychosis, Shaw et al. (2002) again concluded that PTSD symptoms were common and due to both the psychosis itself and adverse events during hospitalization. The subjects with PTSD in this study scored higher on the dissociative items in the Stanford Acute Stress Reaction Ques-

tionnaire, which is consistent with the theory of a dissociative subtype of schizophrenia.

Meyer et al. (1999) found an 11 percent rate of PTSD among forty-
six schizophrenic and delusional subjects. They concluded that 69
percent of the traumatic symptoms were related to the psychosis,
while 24 percent were related to events occurring during the hospitalization. They noted that a high PANSS positive symptom score eight
weeks after hospitalization was the most powerful predictor of PTSD.

Sautter et al. (1999) compared combat veterans with PTSD (N =
22), psychosis (N = 16), and both PTSD and psychosis (N = 24) on a
variety of measures. The individuals with both PTSD and psychosis
reported more positive symptoms than the other two groups, and
more of many different forms of comorbidity. Within the limitations
of the study, the data showed that psychotic symptoms are more characteristic of a subgroup of PTSD than they are of psychotic disorders
without PTSD.

Sautter et al. (2002) studied 82 first-degree relatives of 16 combat
veterans with PTSD who did not have psychotic symptoms; 113 first-
degree relatives of 23 veterans with PTSD and psychotic symptoms;
and 62 first-degree relatives of 15 healthy controls. Using the SCID,
they found one case of a psychotic disorder in each of the three
groups. They concluded that the psychotic symptoms among veterans with PTSD were not associated with elevated rates of psychosis
in first-degree relatives, and therefore were not due to a psychotic
process or disorder independent of the PTSD.

This finding is consistent with my thesis that psychotic symptoms
are a core aspect of the trauma response. If this is true, then antipsychotic medications could be as effective for PTSD as they are for
schizophrenia. No data on this possibility exist. However, Stein,
Kline, and Matloff (2002) showed, in a small study involving nineteen subjects with PTSD who were minimally responsive to an adequate trial of a selective serotonin reuptake inhibitor (SSRI) medication, that olanzapine augmented the response to the SSRI more
effectively than did placebo.

The efficacy of antipsychotic medications in PTSD, if demonstrated, would provide additional but weak evidence in favor of my
theory that psychotic symptoms can be part of a polydiagnostic
trauma response. The evidence would be weak because one cannot

infer etiology from response to medication in psychiatry, and because the different classes of medication are equally effective for an ever-expanding circle of diagnostic categories. The increasing number of FDA-approved indications for SSRIs, for instance, points to the lack of biological differences between the DSM-IV-TR categories of anxiety disorders, eating disorders, and mood disorders, a list to which we can probably add personality disorders and impulse-control disorders.

Similarly, the expanding role of mood stabilizers in treatment of schizophrenia argues against schizophrenia being biologically distinct from mood disorders. Citrome et al. (2002) reviewed prescription data on 8,405 inpatients with DSM-IV diagnoses of schizophrenia treated in psychiatric hospitals operated by the New York State Office of Mental Health in 1994. Individuals with diagnoses of schizoaffective disorder were excluded. They then reviewed records of 4,139 people treated for schizophrenia in 2001.

In 1994, 26.2 percent of people treated for schizophrenia received a mood stabilizer, while 47.1 percent received this class of medication in 2001; in 2001, 59.1 percent of inpatients received a mood stabilizer irrespective of diagnosis. The largest growth was in prescriptions for valproate. I predict that the majority of mood stabilizer prescriptions for people with schizophrenia are written for those who meet criteria for the dissociative subtype. Mood stabilizers are also used clinically in treatment of PTSD and DID, which provides additional evidence for an overlap between these categories; PTSD overlaps with and is highly comorbid with depression.

Lysaker et al. (2001) studied the relationship between childhood sexual trauma and psychosocial functioning among fifty-four adults with schizophrenia, of whom nineteen (35.2 percent) reported childhood sexual abuse. Although they did not inquire about dissociation or PTSD, they found higher neuroticism scores and poorer functioning among the sexually abused subjects. I would expect to find significant rates of PTSD among the abused subjects in this sample.

McGorry et al. (1991) studied thirty-six patients recovering from an acute psychotic episode and found a prevalence of PTSD of 46 percent at four months and 35 percent at eleven months during a one-year follow-up postdischarge.

Mueser et al. (1998) studied trauma exposure and PTSD in 275 patients with severe mental illness, of whom 94 had schizophrenia or schizoaffective disorder and 115 had depression or bipolar mood disorder. In terms of childhood trauma, they found that 44.7 percent reported sexual assault; 18.3 percent physical assault without a weapon; 16.9 percent physical assault with a weapon; 15.6 percent witnessing a killing or serious injury of another person; 7.3 percent the death of a friend or relative by murder or a drunk driver; 14.3 percent a car or work accident; and 8.7 percent involvement in a natural disaster.

The subjects also reported high levels of trauma in adulthood, including sexual assault in 46.7 percent. The overall rate of current PTSD in the 275 subjects was 43 percent: broken down by diagnosis, the rates of current PTSD were 58 percent for depression, 54 percent for borderline personality disorder, 40 percent for bipolar mood disorder, 37 percent for schizoaffective disorder, and 28 percent for schizophrenia. These data are consistent with my prediction that the dissociative subtype affects 25 to 40 percent of subjects with schizophrenia.

Rosenberg et al. (2001), in a review of the literature, found that between 34 and 53 percent of individuals with severe mental illness report childhood physical or sexual abuse, while 29 to 43 percent meet criteria for PTSD. In a particularly severe subgroup, episodically homeless women with severe mental illness, rates of lifetime victimization were 77 to 97 percent. These authors pointed out the paucity of research, funding, and clinical service for psychological trauma among individuals with psychotic mental illnesses, and called for greater awareness of the problem among policymakers, system administrators, and providers.

The Rosenberg et al. (2001) viewpoint contrasts with a typical case discussion and literature review of schizophrenia (Goff, 2002) in which psychological trauma and dissociation were not mentioned. Most of the literature on the etiology of schizophrenia is silent on events occurring after the immediate postnatal period. The environmental variables receiving the most attention and discussion are viral infections in utero and hypoxia during labor; "stress" is mentioned but no data or references on it are to be found in typical reviews and discussions (Goff, 2002).

The literature on PTSD and psychosis supports the postulates and predictions of the theory of a dissociative subtype of schizophrenia.

There are no disconfirming studies in the literature, which is reviewed by Rosenberg et al. (2002).

Bebbington et al. (1993) studied the relationship between stressful life events and onset of psychosis in 52 subjects with schizophrenia, 31 with mania, 14 with psychotic depression, and 207 controls. They found that severe events, involving marked or moderate threat, were more frequent among the psychotic subjects, especially in the three months prior to onset of psychosis. For instance, events rated as moderate or marked threat and occurring in the three months before onset of psychosis for the clinical subjects, or before interview for the controls, were reported by 10.1 percent of 207 controls and 51.9 percent of 52 subjects with schizophrenia.

In contrast, between four and six months prior to the onset of psychosis, or prior to interview for the controls, severe events were reported by 10.1 percent of controls and 26.9 percent of schizophrenia subjects. People with schizophrenia have a higher baseline rate of trauma than the general population and experience an increase in trauma prior to the onset of psychosis. Presumably, if the authors had measured PTSD symptoms as well, those symptoms would have increased at the same time as the psychotic symptoms.

The Bebbington et al. (1993) study supports my thesis that psychotic symptoms are often part of the trauma response. The role of psychological trauma in schizophrenia is complex and multifaceted. Trauma can be a predisposing, perpetuating, and precipitating factor in psychosis. Psychosis itself can be traumatic, and psychotic individuals are assaulted, robbed, homeless, and victimized in many ways. Also, unhappily, the treatment provided by the mental health system can be traumatic.

A PROSPECTIVE STUDY OF THE DISSOCIATIVE SUBTYPE OF SCHIZOPHRENIA

In order to determine whether the dissociative subtype of schizophrenia could be identified in a new sample of patients in treatment for stable, long-term DSM-IV-TR diagnoses of schizophrenia, I (Ross and Keyes, unpublished data) administered the DES, the DDIS, the SAPS (Andreasen, 1984), and the SANS (Andreasen, 1983) to sixty individuals in central Florida. Since these data are under review and have not yet been accepted for publication, they should be given less weight than a published study.

The sixty schizophrenic subjects in the Florida sample did not differ from eighty-three subjects in a previous sample (Ross, Anderson, and Clark, 1994) on age, sex, DES scores, percentage with sexual and/or physical abuse on the DDIS, or the number of secondary features of DID, positive amnesia items, or Schneiderian first-rank symptoms of schizophrenia on the DDIS. They therefore did not appear to be an unusual sample with respect to trauma, dissociation, and positive symptoms.

On an a priori basis, I elected to divide the sample into two groups: scores under 10 on the DES and no dissociative disorder on the DDIS, and scores above 25 on the DES and/or a dissociative disorder on the DDIS. I assumed that there would be a group of intermediate subjects who would be dropped from the analysis based on these criteria. It turned out, however, that no subjects were lost from the analysis because no one with DES scores between 10 and 25 failed to meet criteria for a dissociative disorder on the DDIS.

All study variables conformed to the predictions of the theory of a dissociative subtype of schizophrenia, with one exception—the dissociative schizophrenia subjects in the Florida sample had more negative symptoms than the nondissociative group. The theory predicts that subjects with dissociative schizophrenia will have fewer negative symptoms than those with nondissociative subtypes. This was true in the study by Ellason and Ross (1995). To date, negative symptoms are the only variable with inconsistent findings across different studies; the theory may require revision concerning negative symptoms in the future.

The trauma histories of the high and low dissociators in the Florida sample are shown in Table 11.14. Duration of abuse did not differ between the two groups; this means that low-dissociation subjects with trauma histories had the same duration of physical or sexual abuse as those in the high-dissociation group. However, far fewer subjects reported abuse in the low-dissociation group. Since the number of perpetrators of both physical and sexual abuse, and the number of types of sexual abuse reported, were all greater in the high-dissociation group, the data indicate that their trauma was more severe overall than that of the low dissociators.

TABLE 11.14. Trauma histories of high- and low-dissociation subgroups within schizophrenia

Abuse variable	High dissociation (N = 36)	Low dissociation (N = 24)	p
Sexual abuse (%)	56	13	.005
Physical abuse (%)	50	17	.03
Physical and/or sexual abuse (%)	67	21	.003
Duration of sexual abuse (years)	7.7	6.3	NS
Number of perpetrators of sexual abuse	1.3	0.3	.005
Number of types of sexual abuse perpetrated	2.4	0.5	.009
Duration of physical abuse (years)	14.7	10.7	NS
Number of perpetrators of physical abuse	1.5	0.2	.01

The DDIS (Ross, 1997; <www.rossinst.com>) includes a list of possible perpetrators of physical abuse, and the same list is repeated in the section on sexual abuse. Possible abusers include father, mother, male relative, female relative, etc. The number of perpetrators is the number of these categories endorsed by the respondent.

The DDIS, SAPS, and SANS symptom profiles of the two groups are shown in Table 11.15. As predicted by the theory, the dissociative subjects had more comorbidity and also more positive symptoms of schizophrenia. That is, they were more schizophrenic than the nondissociative subjects based on DSM-IV-TR, Schneiderian, and SAPS criteria. The positive symptoms cannot be a form of comorbidity in schizophrenia because they are the operationalized essence of the disorder.

Negative symptoms as measured by the SANS were also more common in the nondissociative group, but the difference between the two groups was not as striking as it was for positive symptoms. Future studies should include both the PANSS and the SAPS and SANS in order to determine the rate of agreement, or disagreement, between

TABLE 11.15. Symptom profiles of high- and low-dissociation subgroups within schizophrenia

DDIS symptom cluster	High dissociation (N = 36)*	Low dissociation (N =24)*	p
Somatic	11.0	5.8	.0008
Borderline criteria	5.9	2.6	.00001
ESP/paranormal experiences)	4.9	1.8	.0001
Schneiderian	5.0	1.3	.0001
SAPS**	50.7	25.1	.0001
SANS**	38.0	23.4	.04

Note: DDIS = Dissociative Disorders Interview Schedule; SAPS = Scale for Assessment of Positive Symptoms; SANS = Scale for Assessment of Negative Symptoms

* average number of symptoms

** average scores

the three measures. The inconsistent findings for negative symptoms could be due to the measures rather than true variability in the samples.

The Axis I diagnoses made by the DDIS are shown in Table 11.16. Somatization disorder was equally common in the two groups only because it has such a low baseline frequency in schizophrenia, and because of the complex algorithm required by the DSM-IV-TR to make the diagnosis. Somatic symptoms are far more common in the dissociative subtype, as shown in Table 11.15. With large or pooled samples, the rate of somatization disorder would probably become statistically different in the two groups.

The data reviewed in this chapter, as well as the numbers in Table 11.16, suggest that substance abuse is equally common in schizophrenia and DID. This pattern persists when schizophrenia is subdivided into high- and low-dissociation groups. It will probably prove to be a true and consistent finding as more studies are conducted.

Sixteen out of the sixty subjects (26.7 percent) were positive for DID, which is consistent with previous studies reported in this chapter. The much higher rate of borderline personality in the dissociative subtype of schizophrenia is consistent with the core role of borderline personality disorder in the trauma model (Ross, 2000b). The higher

TABLE 11.16. Axis I and II profiles of high- and low-dissociation subgroups within schizoprenia

Diagnosis	High dissociation (%) (N = 36)	Low dissociation (%) (N = 24)	p
Substance abuse	58	58	NS
Somatization disorder	8	0	NS
Depression	83	46	.02
Borderline personality disorder	81	13	.00001
Dissociative identity disorder	44	0	.004

rate of depression indicates that the depression is not secondary simply to meeting DSM-IV-TR criteria for schizophrenia.

Depression undoubtedly has numerous causes among people in general, and among people with schizophrenia. Whatever those causes might be, depression appears to be more common in the dissociative subtype of schizophrenia.

The data reviewed in this chapter support the existence of a dissociative subtype of schizophrenia. Psychosis itself, in my opinion, is a major stressor and meets criterion A for PTSD, which is the stressful event. Psychosis threatens the integrity of the organism and also presents a physical danger, since no less than 10 percent of people with schizophrenia eventually commit suicide. There is no logical reason why trauma could not be both a cause and an effect of psychosis. How often each of these directions of causality operates is an empirical question; the existing evidence supports the conclusion that both can occur.

Several studies document the occurrence of PTSD in reaction to a psychotic episode, and all the existing data indicate high rates of PTSD among individuals with schizophrenia (Lundy, 1992; Lysaker et al., 2001; Meyer et al., 1999; Sautter et al., 1999; Shaw, McFarlane, and Bookless, 1997; Shaw, 2002). It is possible that some of the dissociative symptoms in high dissociators with schizophrenia are secondary to the more severe psychosis these people experience, rather than to other forms of trauma.

Individuals with the dissociative subtype of schizophrenia may have more positive symptoms of psychosis for several reasons: more severe childhood trauma; a greater genetic diathesis to schizophrenia; and a greater genetic diathesis to dissociation. They may also have more dissociation for several reasons: more severe childhood trauma; a greater genetic diathesis to schizophrenia, resulting in more trauma due to psychosis; and a greater genetic diathesis to dissociation.

I include these logical possibilities, which cannot be proven or disproven with the existing data, to illustrate the flexibility in theory required for a dispassionate analysis of genes versus environment in schizophrenia. It is a scholarly error to believe that schizophrenia is predominantly genetic; in principle, it could be equally incorrect that dissociation is caused predominantly by the environment. I don't believe this to be the case because the weight of the evidence is clearly against that conclusion, but nevertheless it is a logical possibility that should be considered.

Chapter 12

Case Examples of Dissociative Schizophrenia

Numerous possible and probable cases of dissociative schizophrenia can be found in the psychiatric literature of the last 120 years, including cases described by Breuer and Freud (1986 [1895]) in their *Studies on Hysteria*. I diagnosed Breuer and Freud's cases as dissociative disorders (Ross, 1997), but some of them would also meet criteria for dissociative schizophrenia. A more recent example is the autobiography *I Never Promised You a Rose Garden* (Greenberg, 1964). Joanne Greenberg's description of her schizophrenia fits Bleuler's criteria for the disorder. Her vivid internal fantasy world corresponds to his criterion of *autism;* her apparent disorder of *associations* I would classify as a creative, playful, and rebellious private language; her *affect* was certainly dissociated from her cognition; and her *ambivalence* about her parents was intense.

Admitted to my trauma program, Joanne Greenberg would receive a diagnosis of DDNOS. Her symptoms included depersonalization, derealization, amnesia, and absorption in an inner world populated by interactive characters who influenced her thoughts, feelings, and behavior (e.g., Schneiderian passivity experiences). Her trauma consisted not of overt physical or sexual abuse but a more subtle failure of attachment, nurturance, and validation by her parents.

August Hoch (1911) provided a lengthy and detailed description of a case that appears to me to meet criteria for dissociative schizophrenia. Of course, one cannot make a definitive diagnosis from a case report. The point of this chapter is to provide additional case material that will help the reader make a gestalt switch from the endogenous biomedical paradigm of schizophrenia to the model proposed here. The reader should look at these cases through new lenses, not reach a definitive conclusion about their diagnoses. In addition, these case examples make the point that dissociative schizophrenia has been present in schizophrenia caseloads for a century.

FROM AUGUST HOCH, MD

Dementia Praecox: A Monograph

The first case is that of a young girl of seventeen, who when seen presented a certain amount of excitement; yet without real distress, she tried the doors, made peculiar statements. She said that some one was in distress, that the country was in trouble, that she was "the center of a good deal." She spoke of explosions and automobile accidents, of fires, and the like,—events of which she had learned from headlines in the newspapers which were lying about; but she did not blame herself for it, as melancholics would. She spoke of electricity being applied to her, said that she felt connected in some way; she heard voices which said, "Stand still," "Get up," "Look out," "Danger." She often would not go to bed, and, without being able to explain it, would violently oppose any attempt at putting her to bed. At other times she would not eat, would not pass her urine, was very insistent that some special patients on the ward should not be there. She often asked what things meant, in fact to anything which was at all obtrusive a feeling of self-reference was attached. She slept poorly and ate insufficiently. The patient presented, therefore, a peculiar impulsive behavior, which was never accounted for by the situation, nor by any obvious ideas; a markedly negativistic attitude at times, hallucinations in the form of voices, electricity, and occasionally visions; ideas of reference, odd acts, the whole characterized by a peculiar lack of transparency and want of connection. (Hoch, 1911, pp. 55-56)

Up to this point in the narrative, the case appears to be one of nondissociative schizophrenia. There is no reason to suspect a role of trauma in her symptoms. However, in the next paragraph, it becomes clear that some of the symptoms are related to a specific traumatic event, namely a rape at age six.

The anamnesis told us that the patient had been self-willed, pedantic, with a great desire for consistency and justice; she was ashamed of her menstruation, but withal fairly natural. At six a boy had intercourse with her, and threatened her if she told about it. At about the age of ten she began to masturbate and worried much about this. When eleven, she one morning woke up frightened and saw Christ on the cross. The night before she had sat at the window listening to men who went by, wondering who they were and whether she would ever meet them. She does not remember any other fancies at the time. In the morning after the vision she worried about her masturbation, and then the episode at the age of six came to her mind and she confessed it to her grandmother. When thirteen and fourteen she used to sit more often at the window at night, losing much sleep thereby, dreaming in the same way as when she was eleven. It is probable—but we can only infer it—that sexual fancies occurred at that time. She worked normally until fifteen, when she became absorbed, could not do her work, and half a year later dropped it all. She was sent to a relative, the place where she had lived till she was six; she became worse, surprised her people by saying that she was in love with a man whom she scarcely knew; she kept watching the house of a physician whom she knew but superficially, thought of him a good deal, as she confessed later; she claimed she saw another man, whom she had seen at her own home, pass daily on a train, saying she recognized him only by his hat. When again at home, near the sea, she saw searchlights, and thought the doctor above mentioned was "in distress," saw a vapor with his face in it. When taken to her family doctor there were two men in his waiting room; she thought they were there to tell the doctor of her masturbation, or about her love for the other physician; she also felt that one of the men was exerting electrical influences on her. In a shoe store she thought she recognized the man who passed on the train, and the shoes she bought she never would wear because they were "charged with electricity." Finally, when she was again sent to the same relatives, she at once became more markedly abnormal, spoke of wires being through the house, of being surrounded by electricity, she refused food, hesitated to pass her urine, wanted things "straightened out," was undecided, and suddenly claimed she was married. (pp. 56-57)

At this point in the case description, it appears that the rape influenced the content of some of the symptoms, but the clinical picture was dominated by the Bleulerian features of autism (self-absorption), associations (her thought disorder), ambivalence (being sexually interested in men, real or imaginary, who were also frightening), and affect (feelings and emotional responses that were disconnected from or out of proportion to current external reality). It is not apparent why I would call this a case of dissociative schizophrenia until Hoch studies the psychological meaning of the symptoms.

This patient could be analyzed even during the active stage of her condition, as it was found that she always quieted down when this was done. In the analysis many of the facts which have been embodied in the history were obtained, as well as the following:

It became clear that the idea of electricity represented a very important part of the picture and furnished the key to the situation. She said that electricity was tried in a way that it should not be tried, and said in the same connection that some one was trying to be near her, and finally that different people were trying to marry her, or were trying something which she did not wish to have tried. At last it was found that the electricity was localized in her sexual organs, and that the sensations were quite unlike electricity, but like the feeling she had perceived during the sexual traumatism in the sixth year. This explained, then, the meaning of these sensations. And then the idea that she felt the electricity in the shoe store, and that the shoes were later charged with electricity, also became comprehensible. Moreover, it was found that these sexual sensations increased when she remained in certain positions for any length of time; hence she heard warning voices, saying "Stand up," "Look out"; they were most pronounced in bed; hence she frequently refused to go to bed, fought desperately when put there. The reason why she objected to the presence of certain patients became clear when it was found that all these were patients who wet their bed; that this, as she said, suggested to her kidney disease; the latter in turn suggested a vaginal examination, which her family physician had made, and this led, therefore, directly to the main trend. The refusal of food found its explanation partly in the fact that the sensations increased after eating, partly in that she had heard her family physician say at one time that meat increased the sexual desire. The voices, the idea that some one was in distress, etc., were invariably traced to one of the men mentioned in the history, and were probably also determined by a projection of her own distress.

I think, therefore, that the case resolves itself into this; we have here a girl who had an early concrete sexual experience. This very probably led her thoughts into the direction of sexual matters to a degree which evidently went beyond the normal tendencies of this sort—and more important to note is the fact that certain reactions all along showed that these fancies were evidently disturbing factors. She lost sleep sitting at the window wondering who the men *were who went by,* whether she would meet them, etc.; in this connection it is interesting that immediately after the first episode of this kind she woke up with fright and had a religious vision, and then worried about her masturbation and her earlier experience with the boy. Then the fact that she was ashamed of her menstruation is of interest, and her growing pedantry, her desire to have things right, may have been, as it often is, a reaction to the feeling of guilt about sexual ruminations.

Finally, there came an absorbed period which was so marked that any objective interest and activity became impossible. And then came that peculiar diffuse rather than specific application of her love to real persons, as is the case so frequently in dementia praecox, and which in itself points to the marked lack of sexual adaptation. She said she was in love with several men whom she merely knew from a distance, and thought she saw them in various places.

Now it is very natural that the original and only sexual experience played a part in her fancies, and when these became dominant the sensations connected with it were represented by hallucinations; this was then a wish-fulfillment; but with it came something like a compensation, something like a feeling of guilt arose and she became stirred up, substituted electricity for sexual sensations, and the whole picture was then made up of these sensations,— of a certain excitement, a feeling of danger with warning voices, the ideas of reference, the shunning of anything which recalled the main trend. In other words, the symptoms were largely grouped around the electrical sensations, while others, such as the hallucinations, "I love you," the seeing of the men, the appearance of the fog with the railroad train, the face, and the like, were phenomena parallel to the sexual sensations, but probably because they were not of such a disturbing character they remained comparatively in the background. (pp. 57-59)

This might appear to be a typical case of nondissociative schizophrenia, up to the point at which Hoch mentions the childhood sexual assault. He then presents an artful analysis of the logic and meaning of the symptoms. Because no antipsychotic medications were available in 1911, Hoch talked with his patient about the meaning of her symptoms and her feelings. Rather than causing regression, escalation, or increased psychosis, the psychological intervention was calming and helpful.

If I were treating this woman, I would look for a series of cognitive errors. I would look for self-blame for the sexual assault. I would assume that sexual arousal had been paired with sexual violation, so that normal arousal became both pleasurable and a dangerous threat. I would talk to her about the "electricity" being, along with her menses, normal, healthy bodily functioning. If she was religious, I would ask her who designed her body, and who made it capable of healthy sexual arousal, the answer being God. The situation of her assault was abnormal, but her body couldn't have known that—it simply reacted to sexual stimulation the way it was designed to do.

On the other hand, if she did not experience sexual arousal during the assault, I would make a careful behavioral analysis to determine when and how normal sexual arousal became dangerous "electricity." A host of cultural, family dynamic, and other factors might be identified as contributors to the clinical picture.

I would point out to her how her choice of vocabulary—"electricity"—transforms her normal sexual arousal into a frightening alien force and symptom of insanity. I would recommend changing the vocabulary, which would decatastrophize her reaction to her own body. I would ask what her voices said, and define this as her feelings and conscience talking to her. In short, I would prescribe massive doses of normalization.

The woman's "schizophrenic" ambivalence is a normal, natural, and predictable outcome of her violation: she longs for adult sexual intimacy, which is simultaneously intrusive and frightening. To make sexual intimacy safe, she hides it in fog, fantasies about strangers, and a secret internal world (Bleulerian autism). Men are frightening, powerful, mysterious, attractive, dangerous, intensely interested in her, and indifferent to her. These are comprehensible human conflicts arising from trauma, not simply symptoms of a brain disease.

On the other hand, not all women with childhood sexual trauma meet criteria for schizophrenia in adulthood. Clearly, this woman was in some way predisposed to a psychotic reaction; although her clinical picture includes a lot of nurture, a disorder of nature probably also exists. Therefore I would prescribe both medication and psychotherapy.

If a brain is inflamed or diseased, it doesn't cease to be the organ of the mind or stop producing thoughts, feelings, and perceptions that have meaning and psychological function. The thoughts, feelings, meanings, and functions simply become disordered. The software continues to function but with problems. The core revolutionary assumption of my model is the proposition that repair of software can result in repair of hardware. Psychotherapy can heal a brain damaged by psychological trauma; psychotherapy is a biological treatment. This direction of causality is not allowed by biological psychiatry in its current form, which permits causality to run in only one direction, from brain to mind, in serious mental disorders.

In my model, the brain is not a machine because it has a scientifically demonstrable property not possessed by machines: the brain generates a mind that can initiate and carry out repair of the brain.

FROM SHEILA CANTOR, MD

Introduction to Childhood Schizophrenia

The following vignette from the introduction to Cantor's (1988) text on childhood schizophrenia could be a case of dissociative schizophrenia. Although the description is too brief to reach any conclusions, it could be a case of pure dissociative fugue, with no psychosis. The literature on schizophrenia contains many case examples with similar hints of unrecognized dissociation.

> In July 1973, on the first day of my psychiatry residency, I met my first childhood schizophrenic, a 16-year-old girl whom I shall call "Megan." The chief resident introduced her to me as an "immature personality disorder," explaining to me that she had been admitted in an amnestic state, perplexed, and unable to recall events of the 6 hours immediately prior to admission. The police had picked her up wandering on the streets uncertain of who she was or where she was going. The resident assured me that she was not psychotic and that the entire episode was, no doubt, a variant on an adolescent adjustment reaction.
>
> Megan became my first psychotherapeutic case. In our sessions I experienced myself as being only slightly less perplexed than she was. I tried to explain my concern to my supervisor: I believed that if I pushed her at all she would decompensate into psychosis; he challenged me to do just that, assuring me that it was my own naivete and inexperience that made me so fearful. I pushed her; she dropped out of therapy and returned to the hospital 8 months later floridly psychotic. In the next 15 months she began the arduous task of teaching me how to work with schizophrenic adolescents. (Cantor, 1988, p. 1)

In my opinion, an onset of psychosis in childhood increases the likelihood of an unrecognized dissociative disorder or dissociative schizophrenia, especially if there are auditory hallucinations. The initial fugue in Cantor's case may have been a symptom of DID and the subsequent "floridly psychotic" mental state may have been due to Schneiderian symptoms in a case of DID or dissociative schizophrenia. The case description is too brief to reach any diagnostic conclusions, but the girl presented initially with florid dissociative symptoms. I regret that I never interviewed Cantor's child patients or collaborated with her when we were both in the Department of Psychiatry at the University of Manitoba. I might have learned a lot from them.

The journal *Schizophrenia Bulletin* contains a section called First Person Account. The purpose of the section is to educate professional readers about "the issues and difficulties confronted by consumers of mental health care." Also, the editors

> hope that these accounts will give patients and families a better sense of not being alone in confronting the problems that can be anticipated by persons with serious emotional difficulties. We

welcome other contributions from patients, ex-patients, or family members. Our major editorial requirement is that such contributions be clearly written and organized, and that a novel or unique aspect of schizophrenia be described, with special emphasis on points that will be important for professionals. (Greenblat, 2000, p. 243)

Cases of dissociative schizophrenia are not difficult to find among the first-person accounts in the *Schizophrenia Bulletin*. They are important because they have been reviewed and edited by experts in schizophrenia and are not regarded as questionable cases with uncertain diagnoses. This is what schizophrenia looks like, according to psychiatrists specializing in the disorder.

FROM PATRICIA J. RUOCCHIO

First-Person Account: Fighting the Fight—
The Schizophrenic's Nightmare, Schizophrenia Bulletin

Patricia Ruocchio (1989, 1991) wrote two accounts of her illness for the *Schizophrenia Bulletin*. If I included the following autobiographical description of her symptoms in a book about dissociative disorders or read her account out loud in a workshop or lecture about DID, it would easily pass as a typical case of DID. The disorder Patricia Ruocchio (1989) describes is one of conflict between dissociated personality states.

I have never fought a fight harder than the fight my mind fights against itself. I have two equally tenacious parts of my mind that are often at odds with one another. I go back and forth endlessly, never able to resolve the struggle, because I do not know which part is true. It takes all my energy to keep vacillating and watch the battle being played out. I can almost see it visually. I see one side arguing with the other; the two are diametrically opposed and each side is equally strong. To me, each of these struggles is the fight of my life; to my therapist, it is something I suffer from called "ambivalence."

During these fights, I can be thinking one thing, but then when the antagonistic thought comes in, I can actually feel my brain split. Sometimes it feels as though one part is the good part that punishes the bad part and causes me pain. Sometimes one part seems to censor what the other is allowed to feel. One part is a victim of The People in my head; the other part joins with my therapist in fighting them. What is similar about all these dichotomies is that they basically separate the part of me that is real from the part that is unreal: it is a battle between sanity and insanity.

When my brain is pulled together I feel "solid." I can literally feel my feet on the ground, and I can feel that my thinking is clear. This state occurs rarely. When I am crazy, the insane part takes over. I am a victim of delusion, unreal thoughts, and severe disorganization. I have some sorts of hallucinations and many visual and auditory distortions. When I am in the former state, I feel good but tenuous, waiting for it all to fall apart any minute. The latter state may be terrifying or perhaps tolerable in a neutral kind of way, even if it is uncomfortable. The state that is most unbearable and causes me the most pain is the state in-between.

I am in this state almost all the time, and usually it feels like a vague confusion, a swirling mass of thoughts and images going on in my head and clouding my thinking and functioning. When it speeds up and gets out of control, I get psychotic. When it slows down, I can see the two parts clearly, and it is almost as though I am in a clear phase except that I am at the mercy of my brain and I go tortuously back and forth, believing both parts and feeling torn apart. This causes great pain as my very self, all that I am inside, is rent in pieces.

Usually I feel so torn because one part is a crazy ideation that makes perfect sense in my system of thought and the other part is my observing ego, connected with reality, trying to put a check on unreal thinking. It is as though I am trying to heal myself, but find the crazy side resistant to the intellectual side. Sometimes one side wins, and I begin to think clearly again. Sometimes the other wins, and I get psychotic—a system of delusion taking over all the reality that I once believed and filling it with false or disorganized thoughts.

The part that is good and seems to punish the other part is the side of me that knows reality and knows I am crazy. I blame myself for not being able to let go of my crazy thinking and "get it right." The good part wants to get well and punishes the bad side for not wanting to get well and instead holding onto falsities. The bad or crazy part, not understanding that these are falsities, feels great pain at the hands of the good part. It is emotional pain, but the kind that is vague and inside, and feels almost physical in the misery it inflicts. Often I am doubled over in pain; usually it is because there is some conflict going on that I cannot resolve.

There also exists another nuance to this self-division: when I have mixed feelings, the "right" side, the rational side, will censor what the other side is allowed to feel without being called bad or wrong. When my therapist goes away, I get furious, but I am not allowed to express my anger in words because the real part of me hears him saying that people do come and go and that he has his own life to lead. The result is that I cannot express my anger except by hurting myself. Though I have worked hard on this and no longer cut myself or burn myself, I fear that if I reveal how truly angry I am, he will stop being my therapist, and so I have self-destructive feelings again. Now,

however, I am learning to talk about my feelings instead of acting on them—
an example of the slow integration of the two parts.

It was only recently that I recognized this censoring mechanism with regard to my therapist's vacations. I slowed down enough to see the two parts
of myself and I heard one part saying that it was angry, while the other part
rejoined with, "No, you can't feel that way; it's not allowed because it doesn't
make sense." This process used to move so fast that it made me crazy, and I
always ended up hurting myself or getting psychotic and ending up in the
hospital. If I was not already in the hospital, I always went in while my therapist was gone or when he got back because my rage caused such intense
turmoil.

When I am working with my therapist, a part of me wants to work to dispel
the delusions while a part of me is frightened and resists. This is particularly
true with The People. When I first began talking about them, after I would tell
my therapist something, I was afraid they would be waiting right outside his
door to ambush me and beat me up. Inside his office I could resolve to be on
his side, and together we would be stronger than they were; but when I was
alone, I felt so vulnerable and often could not hold off their attack. The more I
cooperated with my therapist, the more I put myself at risk. Medication helps
sometimes with The People, and now by working with my therapist and my
co-therapist whom I began seeing two years ago, I have more of a sense that
the three of us are stronger than they are. I still believe they are there, but in
working with two people grounded in reality, I can keep their pain away.
(pp. 163-164; reprinted with permission from the National Institute of Mental
Health)

This autobiographical account matches Bleuler's description of
schizophrenia very closely. Ms. Ruocchio describes somatic symptoms, depersonalization, a divided self, ambivalence, and the encap-
sulation of her "psychosis" in one of the dissociated parts of herself.
She would be a typical patient in my trauma program.

There is a problem with her therapy, as she describes it. Her therapist has aligned with one half of her ambivalence. He has formed a
treatment alliance with her "rational" part-self and is working with
that part-self to suppress and control her "psychotic" self. This approach will increase her internal dividedness and conflict and impede
her efforts at integration. Rather than colluding with her adult, executive self's belief that her feelings are psychotic, crazy, delusional, or
irrational, I would try to learn more about the "psychotic" self. I
would expect it to be a traumatized part-self, dominated by unresolved anger, abandonment fears, and magical thinking.

My first task would be to form a treatment alliance with the "psychotic" self by talking indirectly to her, validating her feelings, and making a commitment to changing the attitudes and perceptions of the adult executive self. I would advise the psychotic self that her previous therapist made a mistake: she, the traumatized child, is not a symptom. She has a right to life just like adult Patricia. I would vow to work with adult Patricia to be more accepting, tolerant, and nurturing toward her feelings, rather than defining them as symptoms of a brain disease and rather than suppressing them with medication.

Aligning with one-half of a patient's ambivalence is a common therapeutic error. A female therapist, for instance, might align with her client's anger toward her father, who was a perpetrator of incest. Commonly, a therapist will align with a battered wife's anger toward her husband. The problem is the disavowed other half of the ambivalent feelings. The incest survivor secretly longs for reconciliation with her father, an apology from him, and a future with the father she never had. The battered wife repeatedly returns to the man she loves, determined to improve her performance so that he doesn't have to beat her again.

Therapy cannot proceed to integration, individuation, autonomy, and health if half the ambivalent feelings are suppressed. The effort at suppression always fails, and behavior is once again driven by the magical thinking of the disavowed, traumatized half of the psyche. I have seen this error many times in therapies for DID. In the case of a person in treatment for schizophrenia, such as Patricia Ruocchio, the therapist's aligment with one part-self follows logically from the biological disease model of her problems: her "psychosis" is due to brain disease and must be suppressed.

FROM BARBARA A. TURNER

First-Person Account: The Children of Madness, Schizophrenia Bulletin

This first-person account (Turner, 1993) emphasizes the negative effects of treatment based on the biological disease model of schizophrenia. Case reports of hysterical psychosis, quoted in Chapter 13, provide additional examples of the negative effects of biological psychiatry, circa the 1960s. More often than it should, treatment for schizophrenia in the twenty-first century resembles these examples of 1960s treatment; it is not simply a problem of antiquated behavior put in the past.

There is a concept in psychiatry called the *least restrictive level of care*. This principle is advocated by managed care companies because it reduces costs, but it is also ethical, humane, and good clinical practice. The idea is that patients should not receive inpatient treatment if they are stable enough for day hospital treatment. They should not be in a day hospital program if they are stable enough for outpatient office therapy, and so on. People should not be made involuntary inpatients if they can be treated on a voluntary basis.

Psychotherapy is a less restrictive level of care than ECT, antipsychotic medications, commitment to a state hospital, and lobotomy. Even if it was merely supportive, psychotherapy for Barbara Turner would have had a better cost-benefit ratio than the treatment she received as a child, because of the high costs of that treatment. These costs included hopelessness and demoralization stemming from a life sentence of incurable, progressive, deteriorating brain disease.

Since I was 8, I had heard voices telling me bad things or silly things, or urging me to hurt myself. My first diagnosis of schizophrenia came at age 12. At that time, I began seeing a psychiatrist and taking medications, neither of which helped the voices go away. Before I was 18 I had seen several psychiatrists, taken what felt like every antipsychotic medication known to medical science, and had bad reactions to all of them. At 17, after a course of 30 shock treatments, the doctors told my parents that I was incurably mentally ill and recommended that I be given a lobotomy and placed on the back ward of the State hospital. My parents took me home instead, where I lay on the couch all day. I had no self-esteem, no hopes, no goals. I had schizophrenia and I was "hopelessly mentally ill."

A year later, I met a man and married him after a few days. I refused to go to any more doctors or take any more meds. I wanted to live a normal married life; normal people don't have to take pills to think clearly and act appropriately.

The voices got worse, but I felt I didn't dare get help or tell anyone about them because that would endanger the facade of normalcy that I was attempting to present. By cutting my arms surreptitiously, I could quiet the voices. . . . My family was horrified when I got pregnant. . . . My husband left soon after our son was born. (Turner, 1993, pp. 649-650; reprinted with permission from the National Institute of Mental Health)

When auditory hallucinations persist despite adequate trials of several classes of antipsychotic medication, this is an indication for a trial of clozapine, according to treatment guidelines reviewed in Chapter 16. Failure to respond to adequate trials of several classes of medication would also be an indication for a trial of psychotherapy, if the assumptions and approaches outlined here were adopted in future treatment guidelines.

Barbara Turner's voices were more effectively quieted by self-mutilation than by medication; this historical fact is a red flag for dissociative schizophrenia. If the voices were fixed, meaningless symptoms of brain disease, there is no reason they should respond to self-mutilation.

FROM JANICE C. JORDAN

First-Person Account: Schizophrenia—Adrift in an Anchorless Reality, Schizophrenia Bulletin

Similar to other first-person accounts, Janice Jordan's (1995) auto-biographical sketch could easily pass as a case history of DID, with a few minor edits. For *delusions* I would substitute *magical thinking,* and for *paranoia* I would substitute *fearfulness.* The question then becomes, what experiences caused Ms. Jordan to be fearful and untrusting? Why did she retreat into an internal fantasy world (Bleulerian autism)? Why did her psyche dissociate into an executive self and an ego-alien controller? Why was the controller so angry and demanding of attention from the adult executive self?

Within biological psychiatry in its current form, none of these questions are worth asking because psychotic symptoms have no psychological meaning, cause, or function.

The schizophrenia experience can be a terrifying journey through a world of madness no one can understand, particularly the person traveling through it. It is a journey through a world that is deranged, empty, and devoid of anchors to reality. You feel very much alone. You find it easier to withdraw than cope with a reality that is incongruent with your fantasy world. You feel tormented by distorted perceptions. You cannot distinguish what is real from what is unreal. Schizophrenia affects all aspects of your life. Your thoughts race and you feel fragmented and so very alone with your "craziness."

My name is Janice Jordan. I am a person with schizophrenia. I am also a college graduate with 27 hours toward a master's degree. I have published three articles in national journals and hold a full-time position as a technical editor for a major engineering/technical documentation corporation.

I have suffered from this serious mental illness for over 25 years. In fact, I can't think of a time when I wasn't plagued with hallucinations, delusions and paranoia. At times, I feel like the operator in my brain just doesn't get the message to the right people. It can be very confusing to have to deal with different people in my head. When I become fragmented in my thinking, I start to have my worst problems. I have been hospitalized because of this illness many times, sometimes for as long as 2 to 4 months.

I guess the moment I started recovering was when I asked for help in coping with the schizophrenia. For so long, I refused to accept that I had a serious mental illness. During my adolescence, I thought I was just strange. I was afraid all the time. I had my own fantasy world and spent many days lost in it.

I had one particular friend. I called him the "Controller." He was my secret friend. He took on all of my bad feelings. He was the sum total of my negative feelings and my paranoia. I could see him and hear him, but no one else could.

The problems were compounded when I went off to college. Suddenly, the Controller started demanding all my time and energy. He would punish me if I did something he didn't like. He spent a lot of time yelling at me and making me feel wicked. I didn't know how to stop him from screaming at me and ruling my existence. It got to the point where I couldn't decipher reality from what the Controller was screaming. So I withdrew from society and reality. I couldn't tell anyone what was happening because I was so afraid of being labeled as "crazy." I didn't understand what was going on in my head. I really thought that other "normal" people had Controllers too.

While the Controller was most evident, I was desperately trying to make it in society and through college to earn my degree. The Controller was preventing me from coping with even everyday events. I tried to hide this illness from everyone, particularly my family. How could I tell my family that I had this person inside my head, telling me what to do, think, and say?

However, my secret was slowly killing me. It was becoming more and more difficult to attend classes and understand the subject matter. I spent most of my time listening to the Controller and his demands. I really don't know how I made it through college, much less how I graduated cum laude. I think I made it on a wing and a prayer. Then, as I started graduate school, my thinking became more and more fragmented. One of my psychology professors insisted that I see a counselor at the college. Well, it appeared that I was more than he could handle, so I quit seeing him.

Since my degree is in education, I got a job teaching third grade. This lasted about 3 months, and then I ended up in a psychiatric hospital for 4 months. I just wasn't functioning in the outside world. I was very delusional and paranoid, and I spent much of my time engrossed with my fantasy world and the Controller.

My first therapist tried to get me to open up, but I have to admit that I didn't trust her and couldn't tell her about the Controller. I was still so afraid of being labeled "crazy." I really thought that I had done something evil in my life and that was why I had craziness in my head. I was deathly afraid that I would end up like my three paternal uncles, all of whom committed suicide. I didn't trust anyone. I thought perhaps I had a special calling in life, something beyond normal. Even though the Controller spent most of the time yelling his demands, I think I felt blessed in some strange way. I felt above normal. I think I had the most difficulty accepting the fact that the Controller was only in my world and not in everyone else's world. I honestly thought that everyone could see him and hear him. It progressed to where I thought the world could read my mind and that everything I imagined was being broadcast to the entire world. I would walk around paralyzed with fear that the hallucinations were real and the paranoia was evident to everyone.

My psychosis was present at all times. At one point, I would look at my coworkers and their faces would become distorted. Their teeth looked like fangs ready to devour me. Most of the time I couldn't trust myself to look at anyone for fear of being swallowed. I had no respite from the illness. Even when I tried to sleep, the demons would keep me awake, and at times I would roam the house searching for them. I was being consumed on all sides whether I was awake or asleep. I felt like I was being consumed by the demons. I couldn't understand what was happening to me. How could I convince the world that I wasn't ill, wasn't crazy? I couldn't even convince myself. I knew something was wrong, and I blamed myself. None of my siblings have this illness, so I believed I was the wicked one.

I felt like I was running around in circles, not going anywhere but down into the abyss of "craziness." I couldn't understand why I was plagued with this illness. Why would God do this to me? Everyone around me was looking to blame someone or something. I blamed myself. I was sure it was my fault because I just knew I was wicked. I could see no other possibilities.

In the hospital, every test known to man was run on me. When the psychiatrist said I had paranoid schizophrenia, I didn't believe him. What did he know? He didn't know me. He was just guessing. I was certain he was trying to trick me into believing those lies. Nevertheless, he did start me on an antipsychotic medicine and that was the first of many drugs I have been given over the years.

The first medicine was Thorazine, the granddaddy of all psychoactive medicines. I have also, at one time or another, tried Mellaril, Stelazine, Haldol, Loxitane, Prolixin, and Serentil, to name a few. These medicines seemed to work for a while, but the symptoms always came back and the side effects were not pleasant. Many times, though, I began to think my medicine was poisoning me, and I would quit taking it. Then, the "craziness" would return in full force. I would usually end up in the hospital and with more medication, doctors would stabilize the psychosis. I tried to commit suicide twice during these periods. I wanted to punish myself for having this devastating illness. The Controller was trying to ruin my life. He was making me miserable. Yet, I clung to him like a sinking ship, even though I felt like I was drowning, slowly but surely.

I was truly blessed when I started seeing my present therapist. I have been seeing him for the past 19 years. He has been the buoy in the raging waters of my mind. I was blessed again when I became the patient of my present psychiatrist. He has been taking care of me for over 16 years. They both have been my saviors. They have not hesitated to try new medicines and new approaches. No matter how bad things have been, they have always been there for me, pulling me back into the realm of sanity. They have saved my life more than once.

In fact, it was through them that I started taking Clozaril, a true miracle drug. It doesn't have half the side effects that the other neuroleptics have, and I have done remarkably well on this medication. The only problem with this medicine is its extremely high cost, which is why most people with schizophrenia are not taking it. Fortunately, my medical insurance covers the high cost of this drug. In fact, my medical insurance has paid for all of my hospitalizations and treatment. Sometimes I get scared that they will drop me, but I choose not to dwell on this fear.

I do know that I could not have made it as far as I have today without the love and support of my family, my therapists, and my friends. It was their faith in my ability to overcome this potentially devastating illness that carried me through this journey. There are so many people with serious mental illnesses. We need to know that we, too, can be active participants in society. We do have something to contribute to this world, if we are only given the opportunity. So many wonderful medications are now on the market, medications that allow us to be "normal." It is up to us, people with schizophrenia, to be patient and to be trusting. We must believe that tomorrow is another day, perhaps one day closer to fully understanding schizophrenia, to knowing its cause, and to finding a cure.

Thank you very much for listening to me. It is my hope that I have been one more voice in the darkness—a darkness with a candle glimmering faintly, yet undying. (Jordan, 1993, pp. 501-503; reprinted with permission from the National Institute of Mental Health)

Within the trauma model (Ross, 2000b), Janice Jordan's self-blame is an example of the locus of control shift; the traumatized child shifts the locus of control from inside the adults in her life to inside herself. Her developmentally normal, egocentric, magical worldview causes her to make an attributional error. The abuse is her fault; she caused it; she deserves it; and the abuse proves she is bad, through tautological reasoning. I would look for the events in Ms. Jordan's childhood and adolescence that caused her to shift the locus of control.

Therapy with Janice Jordan, within the trauma model, would involve reversing the locus of control shift though a combination of education and cognitive therapy; forming a treatment alliance with the controller; learning to understand the goals and viewpoint of the controller; increasing communication and cooperation between the controller and the executive self to meet joint, negotiated life goals; and normalization of symptoms at every turn, among other strategies, tasks, and principles described in my previous books (Ross, 1989, 1994, 1995, 1997, 2000b).

It is self-evident to me that this is a case of dissociative schizophrenia. If it is not self-evident to readers, given the preceding argument and evidence presented in this book, then I am at a loss as to how to stimulate the gestalt switch to my viewpoint.

Janice Jordan's response to clozapine (Clozaril) is consistent with the theory of dissociative schizophrenia. I predict that individuals with the dissociative subtype of schizophrenia are less responsive to conventional neuroleptics than individuals with nondissociative subtypes. To undergo a trial of clozapine, a person must have failed to respond to adequate trials of at least two conventional neuroleptics. It follows, then, that individuals treated with clozapine are more likely to have dissociative schizophrenia.

I predict further that responders to clozapine will be more highly dissociative than nonresponders. If these predictions do not turn out to be true for clozapine, I would still expect them to be true for a medication developed in the future. If the dissociative subtype does have a distinct psychobiology, as predicted by the theory, then it should be possible to develop medications that are selective for these biological differences. I predict that a combination of such medication and trauma therapy will be more effective for dissociative schizophrenia than either medication alone or psychotherapy alone.

FROM LESLIE GREENBLAT

First-Person Account: Understanding Health As a Continuum, Schizophrenia Bulletin

Leslie Greenblat's (2000) description of her gradual recovery illustrates many of the basic principles of the trauma therapy of dissociative schizophrenia. As in the treatment plan for Janice Jordan, the goal would be to help Ms. Greenblat understand that her voices are not symptoms of insanity, demon possession, or brain disease; they are her own thoughts and feelings talking to her. The goal is to make the voices part of the self. They are not the enemy, although they can be critical and even abusive. Abusive voices are self-abuse. If the person were not angry with herself, she would not have voices that are angry with her. Often, the voices are based on identification with the aggressor, which often is one or both of the parents.

It is helpful to redefine the voices as "old tapes," because old tapes can be ignored, taped over, turned off, or discarded. If the voices are old tapes, then a series of questions arises: "Why do you continue to play these tapes over and over in your head? Why do you agree with what they say? What function does it serve for you in the present, to listen to those tapes? Why do you choose to believe that you are helpless to control the voices?"

These questions imply that the person is not insane, not powerless, not a victim of brain disease, and not hopeless. I don't leave those implications unspoken—I actively educate the patient about them. If the endogenous biomedical disease model of schizophrenia is mistaken in a subgroup of patients, then we could withdraw it, and release our patients from a scientifically mistaken life sentence of brain disease.

When I think of my voices as external or separate entities, I find myself demoralized, asking, "Why didn't I think of that?" Sometimes I have a very hard time thinking of these thoughts as mine. When I find myself in this situation, I can be very critical of myself, constantly pushing to be creative and clever. I am, however, coming to understand that what sounds to me like an outside commentary is from my own thinking. So even if I "hear" someone saying, "Look, she's at the computer writing," I can rephrase it to myself, "I am at the computer writing." I shift from third person to first person.

Sometimes it's hard to accept that I generated these seemingly external observations. I avoid the use of "voice" to describe what occurs in my thinking. Instead, I prefer to conceptualize these occurrences by saying it is *as if* I hear "voices." As I move along in my recovery, I am better able to own what I think as belonging to me . . .

I think the quality of the thought-voices evolved as my health evolved. I no longer hear suggestions to run into traffic; if I did, I would refuse. I'm able to judge the appropriateness of the advice. More often than not the thought-voices are reasonable—if nagging. Now they tell me not to eat too many cherries, for example. I hear advice to get enough sleep, eat sensibly, get my exercise. They really bug me about exercise, but I believe it's *me* telling me to get exercise. I'm a thinking, intelligent woman. I know I need to get exercise. But for some reason, I tend to hear it as coming from someone or somewhere else. It's difficult to really concretely define "voices" for someone else. Sometimes it seems they serve as reminders of things I should or shouldn't do—doubts vocalized. (Greenblat, 2000, pp. 244-245; reprinted with permission from the National Institute of Mental Health)

I don't in fact know whether any of the people whose case histories are described in this chapter have dissociative schizophrenia. I don't know whether they are candidates for psychotherapy; they may not be. Their case histories do, however, illustrate typical features of dissociative schizophrenia. The case histories provide an opportunity to explain the principles and strategies I would use in working with dissociative schizophrenia. Based on the information available, I consider all these individuals to be candidates for trauma therapy. Whether such therapy would actually benefit them could only be determined by an empirical trial. This is equally true for a trial of antipsychotic medication; in the individual case, one can only determine whether a given medication works by trying it.

The theory of a dissociative subtype of schizophrenia provides operationalized and scientifically testable indicators for a trial of psychotherapy. No other subtype of schizophrenia performs this function.

Chapter 13

Hysterical and Reactive Psychoses

There was an active literature on hysterical and reactive psychoses thirty-five years ago. Numerous case examples, small case series, and theoretical formulations were published in books and journals (e.g., Hirsch and Hollender, 1969; Hollender and Hirsch, 1964; Kind, 1966; Jauch and Carpenter, 1988a,b; Kantor and Herron, 1966; Mallet and Gold, 1964; Martin, 1971; Richman and White, 1970; Siomopoulos, 1971; Spiegel and Fink, 1979). However, hysterical and reactive psychoses are virtually nonexistent in the literature of the last decade.

Hollender and Hirsch (1964) commented,

> Hysterical psychosis was a popular term in this country and in Europe during the early part of the [twentieth] century. Since the term never became part of the standard nomenclature, many psychiatrists assume that it suffered the fate of other terms once in vogue and now all but forgotten. Yet, it is still very much with us. There is even reason to believe that its popularity today is no less than it was half a century ago. . . . Since no system of classification includes the term hysterical psychosis, it has lived on without official sanction. Standard textbooks do not mention it by name and only by inference can we surmise that it is subsumed under hysteria (as a neurosis). . . . Our search of the literature revealed no article in which hysterical psychosis as an entity was considered. When mentioned in connection with case reports, it received only passing or incidental notice. Since the term is so widely known and used, it seems appropriate to set down how it is used. (p. 1066)

A brief revival of the literature on hysterical psychosis followed this article by Hollender and Hirsch (1964), but the diagnosis disappeared again, receiving almost no academic or research attention after 1979 (Van der Hart, Witztum, and Friedman, 1993). I am persuaded by the argument of Van der Hart, Witztum, and Friedman (1993) that many of these cases were dissociative in nature. I predict that individuals who have received diagnoses of reactive or hysterical psychosis would frequently have high scores on measures of dissociation, extensive comorbidity, and serious trauma histories. This prediction is consistent with case descriptions in the literature. The literature on hysterical and reactive psychoses, then, provides evidence for the existence of dissociative schizophrenia at the level of single cases or small case series.

The treatment literature for hysterical psychosis from forty years ago is somewhat alarming. Mallet and Gold (1964) describe the inpatient treatment of an unmarried twenty-seven-year-old doctor at Guy's Hospital in England as follows:

During the first 4 months she was treated with intensive psychotherapy, and with imipramine and E.C.T. She became increasingly disturbed and unable to utilize the psychotherapeutic relationship. During the next 8 months she received further physical treatment, including high dosages with trifluoperazine, E.C.T. and continuous narcosis; but her condition deteriorated. She described terrible feelings of inadequacy and of 'nothingness, meaninglessness, and a lack of feeling so severe that I cannot be depressed.' She said that people looked like waxworks and that she felt blind and emotionally dead. She developed a strong negative transference for the members of the staff who had been engaged in her treatment. A diagnosis of schizophrenia was made and at her request the patient was transferred to a psychiatric unit in a teaching hospital.

Here she at first received E.C.T., L.S.D. and stimulants. She maintained throughout, as she had at the previous hospital, that treatment would be of no avail unless she could have psychotherapy from the head of the psychiatric department. However, she grudgingly accepted treatment from a registrar who combined psychotherapy with the administration of lysergic acid and cannabis indica. The drugs were regarded by the patient as "an assault on my personality and integrity," and she became more insistent that she could be helped by no one but the head of the department or the superintendent of the previous hospital. During interviews it was clear that the patient was engrossed by the disturbed parental relationship which had marred her childhood. (p. 61; reproduced with permission from the *British Journal of Medical Psychology* ©The British Psychological Society)

This physician-patient may or may not have had dissociative schizophrenia. She appears to have experienced severe depersonalization and derealization, and may have had a traumatic childhood. The purpose of my quoting this vignette is to document the treatment plans often developed for hysterical psychoses.

Treatment outcomes with these methods were not good. In a series of thirteen cases (Mallett and Gold, 1964), "Every patient received physical treatment (including E.C.T., modified insulin, phenothiazines and related drugs in high dosage, or a combination of these) after being diagnosed schizophrenic" (p. 65). Of the thirteen patients, five completed suicide, and the remaining eight had all attempted suicide at least twice while in treatment. When diagnoses were changed to hysterical psychosis, the treatment did not appear to change. Mallett and Gold (1964) commented, "The high incidence of death by suicide was not readily explained" (p. 68).

I have documented the origins of LSD and prolonged drug-induced sleep therapies in my book, *BLUEBIRD: Deliberate Creation of Multiple Personality by Psychiatrists* (Ross, 2000a). If, as I predict, such cases were a significant proportion of individuals in treatment for schizophrenia forty years ago, then it is clear that psychiatry needed to adjust both its countertransference toward this group of patients and its treatment methods. The case just described included prominent symptoms of derealization and depersonalization, both of which would be exacerbated by LSD.

Sedman (1966a,b) described the management of a case of hysterical psychosis at Whiteley Wood Clinic in Sheffield, England. His commentary provides an example of a belittling, hostile countertransference toward a woman likely to meet criteria for DID on structured interview and likely to be in the dissociative taxon on the DES-T (Sedman, 1966a).

Thus, in one patient the presenting complaint was of "blackouts" which were undoubtedly psychogenic. During an interview, if one pursued a line of enquiry which caused her upset, she would suddenly go "glassy-eyed," sit motionless in the chair and refuse to answer. Such a manoeuvre was attempted by the patient during her case conference, but when she was taken to task about it the behaviour ceased. At other times she would adopt an attitude of perplexity, as if she did not know what was happening to her, although, as was subsequently shown, this behaviour was feigned to avoid certain topics of conversation. Whilst she was in the ward, scenes with other patients were frequent, the slightest upset would precipitate bouts of crying or sometimes "black-outs." There was a perpetual clamouring for the doctor or the sister in charge to discuss her problems, though once given the opportunity the real issue would be avoided.

The superficial emotional responses and their exaggerations at convenient times highlighted the attention-seeking side of her personality though this was interwoven with and inseparable from a basic self-insecurity. She had developed a number of phobias and rituals, having been all her life a meticulous, conscientious and house proud woman. She was indecisive, often tense and anxious. Sexually she had been frigid in both her marriages, though she was not above a certain amount of mild flirtatious behaviour in the ward. She would seek to discuss her sexual problems and then adopt a defensive role or shun questions altogether. This ambivalence was apparent in many other aspects, particularly in her interpersonal relationships. Her moods were labile, shifting; tension and anxiety alternating with good humour and somewhat childish giggling, only to be replaced by depression, bouts of crying and stubborness. Following her mother's death this patient developed an experience of being controlled by her mother, who she felt had entered her body. . . . Whatever label one cares to put on such individuals, they are well known to every psychiatric clinic. (pp. 14-15)

Similar to the other cases in this and the preceding chapter, this woman would fit in well in my trauma program. Her dissociative symptoms are all dismissed as manipulation and "hysteria"—that is, the psychiatrist sees only secondary gain and is blind to any primary gain. His "treatment" of the secondary gain consists of simple commands to change her behavior, which I would predict would work for only a short period of time until the intimidation wore off.

Sedman (1966b) quotes a description by a patient with depressive psychosis that could just as well be a description of auditory hallucinations in hysterical psychosis or dissociative schizophrenia, since both are accompanied by high levels of depression:

I've felt that my head has been divided in two, and at times I've felt that I'm my proper self at the back of my head, and these thoughts have all been at the front of my head. . . . It was like my own voice, which you can hear now—it was like that inside my head—other people couldn't hear it because I felt it within me. . . . It doesn't sound as though it's outside—I feel it. I feel as if there is a skin between the front and the back—something I've had to break down. . . . I seem to have a battle between the two parts. (p. 487)

Spiegel and Fink (1979) described a case of hysterical psychosis in an article titled "Hysterical Psychosis and Hypnotizability." They recognized the traumatic origins and dissociative nature of the symptoms, had a positive countertransference, provided individual and family therapy, and reported the patient to be free of psychotic symptoms without medication throughout one year of follow-up. Although this is a single case, it supports my predictions concerning dissociative schizophrenia, a category that would subsume most cases of reactive and hysterical psychosis: the etiology is traumatic, the symptoms are predominantly dissociative, and the outcome is good with positive countertransference and informed psychotherapy. Spiegel and Fink (1979) wrote:

Michael, a 15-year-old boy, was agitated and combative when he was brought to a hospital emergency room. He was placed in four-point restraints. He told the admitting physician that he was "possessed by demons of Satan." Michael reported that when he was lying in bed at home that evening he began to feel "shaky." He was then amnesic for the events that followed until he came to the hospital. His family noted that he began speaking "in a bizarre, awful voice, uttering obscenities, grunting, growling, and sniffing like a wild animal." They became frightened and attempted to hold him down, but he struggled with them. The family reported that he had "superhuman strength" while in this state, and the police were called to help get him to the hospital. (p. 779)

Spiegel and Fink (1979) described the family context, specific traumatic origins, psychological meaning, and function of the symptoms. This approach should be the norm in future studies of the treatment of dissociative schizophrenia.

Chapter 14

Proposed Diagnostic Criteria for Dissociative Schizophrenia

I have designed the diagnostic criteria for the dissociative subtype of schizophrenia so that they could easily be incorporated in a future edition of the DSM. I have used the same format and language as that for the other subtypes. The criteria set is *polythetic* as opposed to *monothetic*. This means that a certain number of items must be present out of a list of items but no items are absolutely required.

The criteria for childhood trauma and extensive comorbidity are not required absolutely to allow for nontrauma pathways to dissociative schizophrenia. There is no reason, in principle, why a dissociative subtype could not be caused by abnormal genes, viral infections, or any of countless other variables. The core of the subtype is the dissociative phenomenology: voices tending to have structured characteristics; voices tending to interact with each other and outside people; and the relative absence of severe cognitive disorganization or thought disorder. Thought disorder can occur on a transient basis due to internal hyperarousal, chaos, and trauma reenactment, but most of the time the individual is lucid and rational.

The option of making an independent Axis I diagnosis of a dissociative disorder is left to the clinician. I set up the criteria in this way because the problem of whether to regard the dissociative disorder as comorbid or as part of the schizophrenia requires further study, discussion, and consideration. Inversely, the clinician can make a diagnosis of a dissociative disorder and not diagnose dissociative schizophrenia if he or she so desires. Future modifications of the criteria sets and text in the dissociative disorders section of the DSM are outside the focus of this book.

The criteria set is designed to cause no disruption to established DSM rules for diagnosing dissociative disorders. There is no point in trying to force changes on the dissociative disorders field by designing diagnostic criteria that abruptly alter established practices. Similarly, the general and subtype criteria in the schizophrenia section of the DSM are left unchanged, except for the addition of the dissociative subtype.

The criteria could be included in Appendix B of a future edition of the DSM, which is called "Criteria Sets and Axes Provided for Further Study." I submit them to the field in general as, in effect, a proposed criteria set for further study.

The DSM-IV-TR (American Psychiatric Association, 2000, p. 313) states, "Because of the limited value of the schizophrenia subtypes in clinical and research settings (e.g., prediction of course, treatment response, correlates of illness), alternative subtyping schemes are being actively investigated." The dissociative subtype of schizophrenia is my contribution to this ongoing active investigation.

295.40 DISSOCIATIVE TYPE

The essential features of the dissociative type of schizophrenia are childhood trauma, extensive comorbidity, and dissociative symptoms. Most if not all individuals meet criteria for numerous other Axis I and II diagnoses including, most commonly, dissociative disorders, depression, post-traumatic stress disorder, borderline personality disorder, obsessive-compulsive disorder, panic disorder, and substance abuse. Most if not all individuals report severe, chronic childhood trauma, which may include sexual abuse, physical abuse, emotional and verbal abuse, family violence, violence outside the family, loss of primary caretakers, and exposure to war, famine, extreme poverty, starvation, natural disasters, and serious illness and disease. Prominent dissociative symptoms include auditory hallucinations, amnesia, depersonalization, and the existence of distinct identities or personality states. The voices often interact with each other and the presenting part of the person; often have specific names, ages, genders, or other characteristics; and often may be engaged in indirect or direct conversation by an outside person. Severe cognitive disorganization or thought disorder is usually absent.

DIAGNOSTIC CRITERIA
FOR 295.40 DISSOCIATIVE TYPE

A type of schizophrenia in which the clinical picture is dominated by at least three of the following:

1. Dissociative amnesia
2. Depersonalization
3. The presence of two or more distinct identities or personality states
4. Auditory hallucinations
5. Extensive comorbidity
6. Severe childhood trauma

The advantage of a polythetic criterion set is that it is not rigid or absolute in its requirement for certain symptoms. Psychiatric disorders are not neat, tidy, and discrete categories. The polythetic criterion set is less likely to impose artificial diagnostic boundaries on groups of symptoms. Polythetic criterion sets tend to be more flexible and open than monothetic ones. Also, polythetic criterion sets in the DSM-IV-TR tend to have more items; therefore they provide a richer description of a given disorder.

The disadvantages of the polythetic criterion set are illustrated by the DSM-IV-TR definition of borderline personality disorder which has nine diagnostic criteria; to receive the diagnosis, one must be positive for five criteria. This means that two people can both be "borderline" but share only one symptom in common. A high degree of variability among members of the same diagnostic category makes it more difficult to establish diagnostic reliability and validity.

Some criteria sets in the DSM-IV-TR are a combination of monothetic and polythetic, such as those for major depressive episode and panic disorder. There is no single pattern in the DSM-IV-TR, which contains multiple examples of monothetic, polythetic, and mixed-type criterion sets. My guiding principle in constructing criteria for dissociative schizophrenia is to be consistent with the format of schizophrenia in the DSM-IV-TR.

PART V:
TREATMENT

Chapter 15

Treatment Outcome Data

In order to be accepted by the field and incorporated in future treatment guidelines and editions of the DSM, the dissociative subtype of schizophrenia must have a replicated, methodologically sound database including studies on diagnostic reliability and validity, biological and psychosocial correlates, and treatment outcome with medication and/or psychotherapy. The psychotherapy must be operationalized in a treatment manual format. Studies must show that it can be taught to therapists, who then deliver the defined protocol to subjects in studies. In addition, studies should include randomization of subjects, a placebo or comparison group, an adequate trial of the treatment, and valid measures of treatment response. Finally, data must show that the treatment works. These are the standard requirements for any diagnosis or treatment modality in medicine.

The only psychotherapy for schizophrenia that approaches these standards at present is cognitive-behavioral therapy (Larsen, Bechdolf, and Birchwood, 2003; Rector and Beck, 2001, 2002). The standards have not yet been met for the dissociative subtype of schizophrenia. To promote the serious study of dissociative schizophrenia, I present treatment outcome data from Ellason and Ross (1996, 1997a). The SCL-90-R data in Table 15.3 are currently under review at a journal. All other data in this chapter were published in Ellason and Ross (1996, 1997a), a systematic, prospective, naturalistic study of treatment outcome for DID.

My purpose is not to prove that there is an effective psychotherapy for dissociative schizophrenia. Rather, my goal is to establish that there are some preliminary treatment outcome data that support the need for future, more rigorous studies. If the preliminary data showed no benefit from treatment, then investment of research resources in trials of psychotherapy would make less sense.

SUBJECTS AND TREATMENT PROVIDED

Subjects (N = 103) in my hospital program in Dallas, Texas, were interviewed with a battery of self-report, computer-scored, and structured interview measures in 1993. They were then interviewed again with the same battery two years later in 1995 (N = 54). At both times, they were asked about symptoms present during the preceding twelve months.

Half the patients in the program come from outside Texas; half are on Medicare disability; and two-thirds meet criteria for borderline personality disorder. They are therefore a difficult group to engage and follow up over a period of two years. There were no demographic or symptom measure differences at baseline between subjects who participated in follow-up and those who did not; therefore the results appear to be generalizable to the population as a whole.

During the two years from 1993 to 1995, the subjects continued to receive outpatient therapy from their referring therapists, after an average inpatient length of stay in my program of about two weeks. No effort was made to control, standardize, or monitor the therapy being delivered but, based on clinical consultations with referral sources, it is generally similar to that described in Ross (1989, 1994, 1995, 1997, 2000b).

I assume that the treatment delivered from 1993 to 1995 was similar to that described in my books for several reasons. The therapists would not refer to my trauma program if they didn't agree with my approach; my approach is consistent with the treatment guidelines of the International Society for the Study of Dissociation (1997) and other authoritative works such as Putnam (1989); the patients describe work with their therapists that is similar to that in my trauma program; trauma program staff often consult directly with referring therapists, and report treatment approaches by those therapists that are similar to ours; our treatment model is similar to that described in a survey of therapist practices (Putnam and Loewenstein , 1993); and no radically different treatment model for DID exists in the literature.

I also assume that the treatment for DID provided from 1993 to 1995 differed significantly from the cognitive therapy for schizophrenia described by Rector and Beck (2001, 2002). Beck's cognitive therapy of schizophrenia resembles the classical cognitive therapy of depression (Beck et al., 1979). For most practitioners, the therapy of DID is more psychodynamic in nature and more technically eclectic than pure cognitive therapy.

METHODOLOGICAL LIMITATIONS OF THE STUDY

The study has both strengths and weaknesses. Its strength is that it is a study of real-world outcomes achieved by therapists in actual clinical settings. The measures used in the study are all valid and reliable, and they were sensitive to treatment outcome. Also, the measures included self-report questionnaires, a computer-scored inventory, and interview-administered structured interviews. Possible interviewer bias was not present for the self-report and computer-scored measures.

The study had a number of weaknesses. The therapy was not structured according to a defined protocol and therefore cannot be rigorously replicated. There was no control group, no randomization, and no comparison treatment. The study therefore corresponds to an open-label medication study with no blind, no randomization, and no placebo group. We did not tabulate antipsychotic medications separately, but overall the subjects were on fewer medications at lower dosages on follow-up than they had been at baseline.

It is a weakness of the study that we did not track medications in detail. In my clinical experience, about 20 percent of patients in the trauma program are on a novel antipsychotic and over 90 percent are on an SSRI antidepressant. In a future study, it will be important to tabulate and track medications carefully. This would be a first step in trying to determine the contribution of various elements of the multi-modal treatment package to symptom reduction.

The only other published prospective treatment outcome study for dissociative disorders is Ross and Ellason (2001). In that study, subjects in my trauma program showed significant score reductions on a number of self-report measures. The measures were administered on admission to the program and again at discharge; average length of stay in the program was eighteen days, including inpatient treatment and step-down to partial hospitalization. Significant score reductions included the psychoticism subscale of the SCL-90-R ($p < .0001$). Scores on the DES did not change in this study. Ellason and Ross

(1996, 1997a) and Ross and Ellason (2001) are the only prospective treatment outcome studies for dissociative disorders available in the literature. Other treatment studies are reviewed in Ross (1997).

LIMITATIONS OF THE LITERATURE

The American Psychiatric Association's "Practice Guideline for the Treatment of Patients with Schizophrenia" (Herz et al., 1997) contains sixteen pages on pharmacological treatments and only half a page on individual therapy. The section on pharmacological treatments spans references 79 to 255, while that on individual therapy includes fifteen references. Dates of publication of these fifteen references, in the order they are cited, are 1968, 1972, 1972, 1973, 1976, 1974, 1974, 1984, 1984, 1980, 1984, 1990, 1995, 1977, and 1988.

Only three of these articles were published in the last sixteen years (McGlashan and Nayfack, 1998; Lehman, Thompson, et al., 1995; Mueser and Berenbaum, 1990). McGlashan and Nayfack (1988) deals with a single case. Mueser and Berenbaum (1990) reviewed the literature on psychodynamic treatment of schizophrenia and identified 159 articles describing treatment of patients with schizophrenia published between 1966 and 1985. They concluded that (1) there is no compelling evidence that psychodynamic psychotherapy of schizophrenia has any efficacy, and (2) there is weak evidence that it is actively harmful.

Lehman, Thompson, et al. (1995) introduced a series of articles on schizophrenia that reviewed psychological interventions (Scott and Dixon, 1995b), family interventions (Dixon and Lehman, 1995), vocational rehabilitation (Lehman, 1995), and assertive community treatment and case management (Scott and Dixon, 1995a). They concluded (Lehman, Carpenter, et al., 1995) that there is no evidence for the efficacy of psychological interventions, other than social skills training. They found that family interventions and assertive community treatment and case management reduce relapse.

The literature on outcomes for the psychotherapy of schizophrenia is tiny and outdated compared to the research funded by drug companies. Rigorous data on psychopharmacology exist because of the profit motive of drug companies, combined with government requirements that adequate studies be submitted before a medication can be sold. If similar multibillion-dollar profit and regulatory incentives applied to the psychotherapy of psychiatric disorders, then we would have a comparable literature on psychotherapy. The difference in size and methodology of the two literatures is driven by capitalism, not by clinical needs or realities. I mention these considerations to set a context for the treatment outcome data presented in the next section.

The data presented have serious limitations. However, they should be evaluated in the context of the existing literature on psychological treatments of schizophrenia. The data, in my opinion, are striking enough to warrant investment of significant resources in future, more rigorous studies.

TREATMENT OUTCOMES

Out of the fifty-four subjects who participated at follow-up, thirty-six (66.7 percent) met criteria for schizophrenia or schizoaffective disorder at baseline according to the SCID (Spitzer et al., 1990). In Tables 15.1, 15.2, and 15.3, I present treatment outcome data on these thirty-six subjects (Ellason and Ross, 1996, 1997a). All would meet the proposed diagnostic criteria for dissociative schizophrenia.

Table 15.1 shows the Axis I and II profiles of the subjects on the SCID. At follow-up, three-quarters of the subjects had been in remis-

TABLE 15.1. Two-year prospective follow-up on subjects with schizophrenia and schizoaffective disorder (N = 36): Active diagnoses on the Structured Clinical Interview for DSM-III-R in the year preceding interview

	1993	1995	Chi-square	*p*
Schizophrenia or schizoaffective disorder	100%	26.5%	25.0	.001
	1993	**1995**	*t*	*p*
Average number of diagnoses positive				
Axis I	5.7	3.0	6.7	.0001
Axis II	3.5	2.3	2.5	.02

Source: Adapted from Ellason and Ross, 1997a.

sion throughout the previous year. A similar reduction in active psychopathology occurred all across Axis I and II. The likelihood that the reduction in psychotic symptoms was due to psychotherapy, and not simply spontaneous remission, regression to the mean, or similar considerations, is increased by the parallel reduction in symptoms on Axis II. It is not plausible that this much spontaneous remission occurred on Axis II, given the quantity of Axis II pathology present at

TABLE 15.2. Two-year prospective follow-up on subjects with schizophrenia and schizoaffective disorder (N = 36): Average number of symptoms positive on the Dissociative Disorders Interview Schedule in the year preceding interview

	1993	**1995**	*t*	*p*
Schneiderian symptoms	6.7	3.9	5.3	.0001
Somatic symptoms	18.2	10.4	6.5	.0001
Secondary features of DID	11.8	8.5	5.8	.0001
Borderline criteria	5.7	3.4	5.1	.0001
ESP/paranormal experiences	6.9	3.2	8.4	.0001

Source: Adapted from Ellason and Ross, 1997a.

Note: DID = dissociative identity disorder

TABLE 15.3. Two-year prospective follow-up on subjects with schizophrenia and schizoaffective disorder (N = 36): Average scores on additional measures

	1993	**1995**	*t*	*p*
PANSS positive symptoms	24.4	16.4	9.7	.0001
PANSS negative symptoms	17.2	13.4	5.3	.0001
Dissociative Experiences Scale	54.5	32.8	5.8	.0001
Beck Depression Inventory	32.7	21.2	3.9	.0006
Hamilton Depression Scale	41.8	25.6	5.2	.0001
SCL-90 global severity index	2.2	1.6	2.9	.009
SCL-90 psychoticism	2.3	1.4	4.1	.0005

Source: Adapted from Ellason and Ross, 1997a.

Note: PANSS = Positive and Negative Syndrome Scale; SCL-90 = Symptom Checklist = 90

baseline (an average of 3.5 DSM-III-R personality disorders per subject). The reduction in Axis II symptoms is likely to be a treatment effect.

Zanarini et al. (2003) followed 275 subjects with borderline personality disorder for six years. During this time, the subjects received active psychotherapeutic treatment. At two years, 34.5 percent of subjects were in remission; at four years, 49.4 percent were in remission; and at six years, 68.6 percent were in remission. This was a naturalistic study without randomization or controls, but it provides evidence that good outcomes can be achieved with borderline personality disorder. Given the high degree of comorbidity between borderline personality disorder, DID, and dissociative schizophrenia (see Chapter 11), the results of Zanarini et al. (2003) suggest that the findings at two years in my study may be valid.

The DDIS findings are shown in Table 15.2. They follow the pattern seen on the SCID in that there is significant symptom reduction on both Axis I and II, and a reduction in psychotic symptoms. Psychotic (Schneiderian) symptoms were reduced by 41.8 percent.

The data in Table 15.3 confirm the general reduction in symptoms all across Axis I and II on a variety of other measures. The reduction in psychotic symptoms is consistent on the SCID, DDIS, PANSS, and SCL-90. In Table 15.4, the Millon Clinical Multiaxial Inventory-II (MCMI-II) (Millon, 1977) is added to this list of measures.

In both clinical and research settings, when testing the efficacy of a medication, it is essential to conduct an *adequate trial*. Criteria for an adequate trial include subjects who meet diagnostic criteria for an appropriate disorder; symptoms that are specified and measured repeatedly in a reliable manner; adequate dosage; and adequate duration of the trial. In other words, the drug has to be given a fair chance to work. No one would reject the use of quetiapine in treatment of schizophrenia if a study showed it had little effect after four days.

Two years is not an adequate trial of the psychotherapy of either DID or dissociative schizophrenia. The duration should be at least five years because the recovery process takes at least that long for most people. Fortunately, however, in this naturalistic prospective study, a subset of subjects did receive an adequate trial of psychotherapy, because subjects were recruited into the study at varying times in the recovery process. Some had received only a few months of psy-

TABLE 15.4. Two-year prospective follow-up on subjects with dissociative identity disorder (DID) who reached integration (N = 12)

Measure	1993	1995	t	p
Dissociative Experiencse Scale	50.5	15.4	8.0	.00001
DDIS Schneiderian	6.2	1.4	5.7	.0001
DDIS somatic symptoms	14.3	4.3	5.8	.0001
DDIS borderline	5.9	1.7	7.0	.00001
DDIS secondary features of DID	11.2	4.1	6.4	.0001
DDIS ESP/paranormal experiences	5.8	1.9	4.6	.0008
DDIS substance abuse	1.3	0.0	4.0	.002
SCID Axis I and II diagnoses	11.5	1.9	7.6	.0001
Beck Depression Inventory	27.9	9.7	4.0	.004
Hamilton Depression Scale	36.5	16.0	4.2	.002
MCMI-II schizoid	25.5	16.5	2.6	.05
MCMI-II schizotypal	71.9	51.1	4.7	.01
MCMI-II paranoid	29.4	18.6	2.5	.05
MCMI-II thought disorder	26.1	8.5	3.3	.01
SCL-90 global severity index	1.95	0.71	5.8	.0004
SCL-90 paranoid ideation	1.72	0.47	4.36	.002
SCL-90 psychotism	1.97	.037	5.72	.0004

Source: Adapted from Ellason and Ross, 1997a.

Note: DDIS = Dissociative Disorders Interview Schedule; MCM-II = Millon Clinical Multiaxial Inventory-II; SCID = Structured Clinical Interview for DSM-III-R; SCL-90 = Symptom Checklist-90.

chotherapy for DID, while others had been in active specific treatment for years. We did not tabulate the duration of prior psychotherapy, unfortunately, which is another limitation of the study.

Because some subjects were further along in their recovery at the time of entry into the study, they received a more adequate treatment trial, as they had received much of their treatment prior to enrollment. In design terms, it would be better to enroll all subjects at the time of initial diagnosis and follow them prospectively for ten years. As this was not possible due to limitations in funding, the best available data on a full trial of treatment are those for twelve subjects who reached stable integration of their DID by the time of follow-up. These twelve subjects received a full trial of treatment by definition, since the goal of treatment is integration.

Integration was defined as follows: the treating therapist confirmed the subject was integrated; the subject agreed he or she was integrated; the subject no longer met criteria for DID on the DDIS; and the subject met five out of Kluft's (1984, 1985) six operationalized criteria for integration. We did not require the presence of the fifth criterion because it is difficult to operationalize. We did not obtain information on the psychotherapy techniques or medications prescribed to the twelve individuals who reached integration.

Kluft's criteria for integration are

1. continuity of contemporary memory,
2. absence of overt behavioral signs of multiplicity,
3. a subjective sense of unity,
4. absence of alter personalities on hypnotic reexploration,
5. modification of transference phenomena consistent with the bringing together of personalities, and
6. clinical evidence that the unified patient's self-representation included acknowledgment of attitudes and awareness previously segregated in separate personalities.

The treatment outcome for DID patients treated to stable integration is excellent. The twelve subjects who reached stable integration had an average of 6.2 Schneiderian symptoms at baseline, which is far above the average for schizophrenia. I am confident they would all have met criteria for dissociative schizophrenia at baseline because they had such high levels of both psychotic and dissociative symptoms, and because all subjects met criteria for DID and schizophrenia or schizoaffective disorder. All subjects would have dissociative schizophrenia by definition if all cases of DID were included within the category of dissociative schizophrenia.

The average reduction in psychotic symptom scores was 77.4 percent on the DDIS, 66.9 percent on the SCL-90 paranoid scale, 81.2 percent on the SCL-90 psychoticism scale, 35.3 percent on the MCMI-II schizoid scale, 28.9 percent on the MCMI-II schizotypal scale, 36.7 percent on the MCMI-II paranoid scale, and 67.4 percent

on the MCMI-II thought disorder scale. These are clinically and statistically significant findings even on the least sensitive subscales of
the MCMI-II.

In comparison, the reduction in scores on the DES was 69.5 percent, on active SCID Axis I and II diagnoses 83.5 percent, and on active borderline criteria 71.2 percent. These are very robust numbers.
To express it another way, the subjects dropped from two standard deviations above the mean for the general population to within the normal range clinically and statistically on the DES.

Remarkably, there was zero active substance abuse in the year preceding the follow-up interviews in a population two-thirds of whom
were substance abusers. To illustrate the potential importance of
these results, I make a simple calculation. Assume that 30 percent of
individuals currently in treatment for schizophrenia meet criteria for
the dissociative subtype (see Chapter 11 for data to support this estimate). Assume that 50 percent of individuals with dissociative schizophrenia can attain the outcome shown in Table 15.4 (a reasonable assumption based on the outcome data presented in this chapter). Assume that schizophrenia will affect 1 percent of the 300 million people in the United States at some point in their lifetimes. This means
that 450,000 ($0.3 \times 0.5 \times 0.01 \times 300,000,000$) people in the United
States could attain this outcome. If the dissociative subtype affects
more than 30 percent of people with schizophrenia, and if more than
50 percent can attain this outcome, the final number goes up to over
half a million people. Worldwide, if treatment were delivered to all affected individuals, this treatment benefit could be realized by 10 million people.

In future studies, therapy will have to be operationalized and moni-
tored, as in any rigorous psychotherapy outcome study. The data reviewed here do not meet criteria for a definitive or rigorous trial.
However, they provide an argument for investing time, energy, and
resources in the study of dissociative schizophrenia.

Chapter 16

Principles of Psychotherapy
for Dissociative Schizophrenia

While preparing to write this chapter, I reviewed treatment guidelines for schizophrenia prepared by the American Psychiatric Association (Herz et al., 1997), the Patient Outcomes Research Team (PORT) (Dixon and Lehman, 1995; Lehman, 1995; Lehman and Steinwachs, 1998; Lehman, Carpenter, et al., 1995; Lehman, Thompson, et al., 1995; Scott and Dixon, 1995a,b), the Expert Consensus Panel for Schizophrenia (McEvoy, Scheifler, and Frances, 1999), and the Texas Medication Algorithm Project (Miller et al., 1999). As well, I read reviews of these guidelines by Smith and Docherty (1998) and Milner and Valenstein (2002), and reviews of the literature on psychotherapy of schizophrenia by Carpenter (1984), Feinsilver and Gunderson (1972), and Fenton (2000). These materials summarize the thinking of the past three decades.

In addition, as mentioned previously, I participated in an ISPS task force that prepared a detailed response to the recommendations concerning psychotherapy of schizophrenia in the PORT report; the articles prepared by the ISPS Task Force filled the March 2003 issue of the *Journal of the American Academy of Psychoanalysis and Dynamic Psychiatry.*

I am in agreement with almost everything in the published treatment guidelines with two noteworthy exceptions: McEvoy, Scheifler, and Frances, 1999) claim, "We do know that schizophrenia is **not** caused by bad parenting, trauma, abuse, or personal weakness" (p. 74).

The authors provide no references, data, analysis of the literature, or argument of any kind to support this claim. In this book, I present references, data, analysis of the literature, and argument in support of the proposition that bad parenting, trauma, and abuse are major etiological factors in schizophrenia. It appears to me that the viewpoint of

McEvoy, Scheifler, and Frances (1999) has not been arrived at through an analytical, dispassionate, scholarly, or scientific process. Their statement is an ideological assertion, not a scientific or medical fact.

In addition, for this assertion by McEvoy, Scheifler, and Frances (1999) to be correct, "personal weakness" and biological or genetic defect must be separate categories. The endogenous biological disease model is based on an inherent defect in the brain—it may be pleasant to assure the affected individual that his or her brain weakness is not a personal weakness, but it is not logical. One cannot be a "strong" person and simultaneously have a "weak" brain unless the brain weakness has no effect on mental state; if this was the case, though, schizophrenia would not be caused by brain disease.

In order to arrive at absolute certainty concerning any possible etiological factor in schizophrenia–McEvoy, Scheifler, and Frances (1999) are absolutely certain that psychosocial factors play no etiological role in schizophrenia—data are required, in this case, negative findings from relevant, methodologically sound studies of the role of childhood trauma and abuse in schizophrenia. No such data exist in the literature, and abundant data disconfirm their viewpoint. This assertion should therefore be removed from all future guidelines for treatment of schizophrenia.

The second point of disagreement concerns the phase of schizophrenia for which psychotherapy is indicated. I propose that specific intensive psychotherapy for psychotic symptoms should be started in the acute phase and then continued during the early postepisode resolution period and during maintenance treatment. My thesis is that properly designed psychotherapy can be as effective as medication for treatment of psychotic symptoms in the dissociative subtype of schizophrenia, similar to the equal efficacy of cognitive therapy and medication for moderately severe depression. As for depression, a combination of medication and psychotherapy will probably prove to be more effective than either used alone.

The Expert Consensus Panel for Schizophrenia Guidelines (Frances, 1999) provide data to support their treatment recommendations. The data are based on the opinions of fifty-seven experts on medication treatment of schizophrenia and sixty-two experts on psychosocial treatment of schizophrenia. Each expert rated various treatment items on a nine-point scale where 1 equals extremely inappropriate and 9 equals extremely appropriate.

For the severely impaired and unstable patient during an acute episode, psychodynamic psychotherapy received an average rating of 1.4; cognitive and social skills training, 4.0; and medication and symptom monitoring, 8.7. For treatment of the moderately impaired and intermittently stable patient during an acute episode, psychodynamic psychotherapy was rated 1.8; cognitive and social skills training, 3.9; and medication and symptom monitoring, 8.4. For treatment of the mildly impaired and often stable patient during an acute episode, psychodynamic psychotherapy received a rating of 1.9; cognitive and social skills training, 3.9; and medication and symptom monitoring, 7.9.

The Expert Consensus Panel opinion is unequivocal: psychodynamic psychotherapy is absolutely contraindicated during the acute psychotic phase for all patients; cognitive therapy is of possible utility; and medication is absolutely indicated.

The type of psychodynamic and/or psychoanalytic psychotherapy considered to be contraindicated by the panel members is probably similar to the approaches described in Strauss et al. (1980). The cognitive therapy they have in mind is probably similar to that described in Wykes, Tarrier, and Lewis (1998) and Kingdon and Turkington (1994). Although these are reasonable assumptions, I cannot be certain because the therapies are not described in any of the guidelines.

The most favorable recommendations for psychotherapy, naturally, are for maintenance-phase treatment of mildly impaired and often stable patients. For this group, psychodynamic psychotherapy received a rating of 2.9; cognitive and social skills training, 5.7 (SD 2.2); and medication and symptom monitoring, 6.7 (SD 2.5). The standard deviations demonstrate that the level of endorsement of cognitive and social skills training overlaps extensively with the level of recommendation for medication in this subgroup of patients.

The Expert Consensus Panel for Schizophrenia endorses the proposition that for a subgroup of patients in one phase of their illness, cognitive therapy is indicated to about the same degree as medication. This means that the treatment perspective in this book is consistent with accepted guidelines for maintenance treatment of mildly impaired and often stable patients with schizophrenia. The difference is that I believe that psychotherapy is also indicated in the acute psychotic phase of schizophrenia. Individuals with the dissociative subtype of schizophrenia may be in the mild, moderate, or severe categories of impairment; therefore my opinion diverges widely from consensus guidelines concerning severe patients in the acute phase of psychosis.

On the other hand, for individuals with nondissociative subtypes of shizophrenia, I agree with the consensus guidelines. It is clear to me that psychodynamic psychotherapy with severe patients in the acute psychotic phase of nondissociative schizophrenia is absolutely contraindicated. This book defines a subgroup of patients for whom treatment guidelines could be modified in the future, pending the outcome of relevant treatment studies.

PRINCIPLES OF TRAUMA THERAPY

The Phases of Trauma Therapy

Courtois (1999) reviewed current thinking about the psychotherapy of survivors of childhood sexual abuse. Her guidelines are applicable to the psychotherapy of adults with all types and combinations of childhood psychological trauma, which may include sexual, physical, emotional, and verbal abuse, neglect, family violence, violence outside the home, loss of primary caretakers, severe poverty, malnutrition, disease, natural disasters, and war. Trauma treatment has an initial, a middle, and a final phase, which are common to all treatment approaches.

The first stage is stabilization. Basic needs and safety requirements must be met, and a treatment alliance must be formed. Establishing trust and rapport are major goals. For someone with schizophrenia, this phase may involve hospitalization, starting or adjusting medications, finding housing and community support, working on basic grooming and life skills, and similar agenda items. All the standard social work tasks and goals in any model of the etiology and treatment of schizophrenia are relevant at the beginning of therapy.

These early priorities are commonly a focus of treatment in my trauma programs. They are not diagnostically specific and are routinely required in treatment plans for psychiatric inpatients, irrespective of primary diagnosis. The need for basic hierarchy-of-need interventions may be greater in treatment planning for a nonpsychotic battered spouse than for a person with florid active psychosis who has good social supports.

Education about diagnoses and treatment modalities, overcoming denial, and continuing to build a positive treatment alliance and shared treatment goals continue throughout the therapy, but predominate in the initial phase. In the initial phase, the person must make a serious commitment to recovery and the hard work of therapy. Although it is impossible to suddenly relinquish all unhealthy defenses, behaviors, and addictions, the person must make an intellectual commitment to change; otherwise, the work cannot begin.

The therapist and client have to set initial and long-term goals and have to agree on a general philosophy of treatment. The client has to accept the working model of etiology and the basic principles of treatment. The structure, rules, and boundaries of therapy must be set and the client must give informed consent to participation in treatment. Informed consent is not a static, one-time event. Rather, it is an ongoing process that requires repeated review of the costs and benefits of therapy. If a basic working partnership cannot be established, the individual might be better served with a different treatment model.

The initial phase of therapy for an acute psychotic episode in schizophrenia could look radically different from typical contemporary treatment. Mosher (1999) summarizes the excellent outcomes of the Soteria Project and its direct successors. He provides evidence that immediate and two-year outcomes without neuroleptic medication or inpatient hospitalization can be as good or better than those for standard treatment. The approach I am outlining here combines aspects of conventional treatment of the Soteria protocol.

As implemented in a hospital setting, my trauma model resembles conventional treatment in many ways. The basic structure of psychiatric inpatient treatment is in place, for instance. There is a medical record. Treatment staff includes an attending physician, nurses, mental health technicians, and therapists. A DSM-IV-TR diagnosis is made and psychotropic medications are prescribed. Insurance companies are billed for treatment and so on.

However, my trauma program differs from conventional treatment in several ways. Treatment is based on a specific, integrated model that is delivered to all patients in the same way. It includes three hours a week of intensive individual psychotherapy (compared to none in most inpatient settings) and thirty-five hours a week of intensive group psychotherapy. On most inpatient units, there is an hour or two a day of group therapy, usually involving fairly simple skills training.

The Soteria Project (Bola and Mosher, 2003; Mosher, 1999) was designed as a radical alternative to psychiatric hospitalization. No medications were prescribed and all staff were nonprofessional. The atmosphere was homelike, with no structured therapy sessions. The average length of stay at Soteria was five months, compared to twelve days in my trauma programs. Soteria therefore differed strongly from my trauma programs in major ways.

However, the core resemblances between the two are more important, in my view. According to Mosher (1999), Soteria "staff worked gently to build bridges, over time, between individuals' emotionally disorganized states to the life events that seem to have precipitated their psychological disintegration" (p. 144).

Soteria was based on an etiological model that emphasized the role of events in the psychosocial environment. The psychoses of its clients were understood as disordered but comprehensible reactions to trauma and stress. The countertransference was positive and the clients were seen as psychologically troubled rather than as biologically diseased. If the trauma model were delivered in a residential treatment center without psychotropic medications, it would resemble Soteria more than conventional psychiatric hospitalization.

I envision a residential treatment center that incorporates the positive countertransference of Soteria, largely rejects the endogenous disease model of schizophrenia, assumes a limited role for medication, and tracks treatment outcome with reliable measures. The center would differ from Soteria mainly by including individual and group psychotherapy sessions based on the trauma model. I see length of stay as averaging sixty days. Such a facility would have to be financed through some combination of self-pay and a philanthropic foundation.

One element of Soteria I would not implement is the use of nonprofessional staff as the primary therapists. In my experience, providing skilled trauma model therapy requires extensive training, supervision, and experience. It requires both intuitive clinical skill and intellectual knowledge. The trauma model has specific rules, procedures, and strategies that take time to learn. Nonprofessionals could certainly work as support and adjunctive staff, and their roles would be valuable and therapeutic. However, trained, credentialed professional staff would also be required to deliver trauma model therapy.

The middle phase of therapy is where most of the hard work takes place. The tasks, strategies, and goals of this phase are described in my previous writings (Ross, 1989, 1994, 1995, 1997, 2000b). The work involves several basic elements. One must resolve conflicted, ambivalent attachment to the perpetrators of childhood abuse and neglect. Core cognitive errors of self-blame, unworthiness, and dirtiness must be corrected. A great deal of loss, sadness, and loneliness must be felt, processed, and left behind. There is a great deal of work on building more healthy, flexible, adapative coping skills, especially strategies for affect management and mood-state regulation.

A trauma narrative is constructed in which the events of childhood are reevaluated and understood from an adult perspective. Sometimes unhealthy relationships have to end, and the person begins to practice choosing healthier friends and supports. Healthy limits and boundaries must be learned and practiced. During the middle phase, symptoms and diagnoses begin to go into remission.

The final phase of therapy focuses on resolution and consolidation of treatment gains, building more fluid and healthy coping skills, and launching major life projects such as education and long-term relationships. The three phases of therapy overlap a great deal and are not discrete categories.

The anticipated duration of treatment is a minimum of five years. Since the standard treatments for schizophrenia last a lifetime, there is no reason that trauma therapy for dissociative schizophrenia should be short term. As is currently true for trauma therapy of DID and DDNOS, most of the treatment is delivered in outpatient office settings. The purpose of the hospital is acute stabilization and return to a less restrictive level of care. The next step down is either partial hospitalization/day hospital or a residential treatment center, just as it is for eating disorders, substance abuse, and other diagnostic categories.

Trauma therapy for dissociative schizophrenia involves numerous principles, goals, tasks, and strategies that can be found in any contemporary treatment model for severe mental disorders. It is important to understand that the similarities between trauma therapy for dissociative schizophrenia and typical contemporary treatment planning for schizophrenia are numerous and substantial. For instance, if we assume that, in conventional treatment, 50 percent of people with schizophrenia discharged from psychiatric hospitals discontinue their antipsychotic medication against medical advice within two years (a conservative estimate), there would be nothing unusual about 50 percent of individuals in trauma therapy being medication free.

Trauma therapy for dissociative schizophrenia also incorporates many of the principles and procedures of dialectical behavior therapy (DBT) for borderline personality disorder (Linehan, 1993), which is a widely accepted and empirically validated form of psychotherapy. DBT is a form of cognitive-behavioral therapy. It is highly structured and has a treatment manual. The dialectical component corresponds to the "collaborative empiricism" of classical cognitive therapy for depression (Beck et al., 1979). Therapist and client work together as a team to test and change core beliefs and cognitions.

DBT emphasizes a commitment to recovery, containment of affect, limit setting, and skills building. Like the trauma model, DBT uses paradox, humor, metaphor, confrontation, and grounding strategies, combined with with empathy, positive countertransference, and validation. Specific treatment goals are set and specific symptoms and behaviors are agreed upon as the targets of therapy. Some exposure to affect is used in DBT but less than in trauma therapy.

The efficacy of DBT is supported by a treatment outcome study in which twenty subjects receiving DBT improved more than twenty-two comparison subjects who received treatment as usual (Linehan et al., 1991). In a one-year prospective follow-up, the borderline patients receiving DBT had less parasuicidal behavior, fewer days in hospital, and a lower dropout rate. Although the data supporting the efficacy of DBT are limited, they provide further support for the efficacy of trauma model therapy, since the two approaches resemble each other.

Treatment as usual for schizophrenia, in contrast, does not resemble trauma model therapy. Agar and Read (2002) reviewed the records of 200 clients at community mental health centers. They found that 46 percent of the files described physical and/or sexual abuse. However, of the ninety-two clients who had reported abuse, only 22 percent received abuse-focused therapy; abuse was mentioned in only 33 percent of the treatment plans for these ninety-two individuals and in only 36 percent of the case formulations. According to my model, the physical and sexual abuse should be taken into account in 100 percent of case formulations and treatment plans for dissociative schizophrenia, and the number of individuals receiving trauma therapy should be much higher than 22 percent. It will never be 100 percent for logistical, compliance, and patient preference reasons.

Therapeutic Neutrality

I have written at length about the principle of therapeutic neutrality in my books on treatment of dissociative disorders. Therapeutic neutrality is an essential principle in trauma therapy irrespective of diagnosis. Given that delusional thinking is a frequent symptom in all forms of schizophrenia, the requirement for neutrality in treatment of the dissociative subtype is, if anything, stonger than that for other disorders.

Therapeutic neutrality pervades all aspects of treatment. For instance, survivors of serious childhood trauma frequently reenact a variety of roles on the victim-rescuer-perpetrator triangle (Ross, 2000b). They may assume the perpetrator role in relationships to undo the victimization of their childhoods, or they may adopt the rescuer role to undo the failure of their caretakers to rescue them. The therapist can be drawn into these reenactments and act out one of the roles on the triangle in reaction to the behavior of the client.

Therapeutic neutrality with respect to the victim-rescuer-perpetrator triangle means that the therapist attempts to maintain a position off the triangle. The goal is to help the client change the dynamics and behaviors of disordered relationships in the present, which cannot occur if the therapist is trapped in a series of reenactments. Similarly, marital therapy for a couple in which one partner has dissociative schizophrenia would require therapeutic neutrality. The therapist would endeavor not to align or collude with either member of the couple.

In treatment of delusional thinking, therapeutic neutrality means adopting a position of neither believing nor disbelieving the content of the delusion. This is a necessary stance because in many cases, it isn't clear which beliefs are accurate, which are slightly distorted, and which are frankly delusional. Even when a belief is definitely delusional, the therapist may maintain neutrality because confrontation or a direct statement that the belief is false may damage the treatment alliance or cause the client to drop out of treatment. In a cognitive-behavioral format the therapist works with the client in a collaborative and empirical manner to test the plausibility of beliefs and thoughts.

In terms of memory content, therapeutic neutrality again means neither believing nor disbelieving the accuracy of the memories. Most of the time, there is no independent corroboration of abuse memories from childhood; therefore the therapist does not know whether the memories are accurate or inaccurate. Trauma model therapy is designed so that the basic tasks, strategies, and techniques are the same whether the memories are assumed to be mostly accurate or mostly inaccurate. The therapist listens empathically but remains neutral.

Mental health professionals often assume that they have only two options: believe or not believe. The client makes the same assumptions and concludes that if the therapist doesn't actively believe, he or she must be actively disbelieving. This is a cognitive error that can be corrected with education and cognitive therapy.

In fact, I neither believe nor disbelieve. I am actively neutral, which is not a passive or default position. My goal is to sketch in the basic logic and principles of trauma therapy for dissociative schizophrenia, not to provide an adequate or full explication of it. That will require a separate book. I am discussing therapy, specifically the principle of therapeutic neutrality, to support the theory of a dissociative subtype of schizophrenia. It is worth considering psychotherapy for dissociative schizophrenia, partly because a defined psychotherapy is available that is supported by preliminary treatment outcome data.

Recovery Occurs at the Level of Process and Structure, Not Content

The next step in the education of the patient is to explain that recovery occurs at the level of process and structure, not content. Treatment is not about memory content. It is about cognitive errors, false beliefs, and unresolved feelings and conflicts that exist in the present and dominate life in the present.

However, recovery involves the construction of a trauma narrative. There is a great deal of conversation about the past, including traumatic events. The conversation involves intense recollection and painful feelings. However, the purpose of therapy is to change the present and the future, and to create more adaptive, flexible, and healthy beliefs, behaviors, and coping strategies. The therapist can err in one of two directions: spending too much time and energy on memories, with no change in the present; or ignoring the past and engaging in an empty, intellectualized therapy that lacks depth.

The therapy focuses on the present but is informed by an understanding of the past. The conflicts, symptoms, cognitive errors, addictions, and self-defeating behaviors do not exist in a vacuum; they have a historical context. The trauma model, I often say, is a "There but for the grace of God, go I" model. It assumes that the person is exhibiting a biologically and humanly normal reaction to the gauntlet he or she has run, which is the traumatic childhood. The person may have overreacted somewhat based on a diagnostically nonspecific temperament or sensitivity to environmental stress, but he or she does not suffer from an endogenous, diagnostically specific biological defect. I am in full agreement with anyone who believes that temperament is genetically determined.

Trauma therapy does not involve abreaction, regression therapy, or indulging in the victim role or dysfunctional feelings. It does not provide an excuse for bad choices or bad behavior. Nor does it involve blaming problems on others. It involves taking responsibility for addictions, acting out, and destructive behavior, and working hard to make real changes.

The Problem Is Not the Problem

Within the trauma model, all symptoms, mental states, beliefs, and behaviors have a context and a function, meaning and purpose. Clearly, this assumption would not apply to an anticholinergic delirium caused by an overdose of benztropine. I might treat that problem with IV diazepam, reduced environmental stimulation, and nursing observation. Psychotherapy would be useless during the period of delirium.

I assume that both acute and chronic psychotic episodes in dissociative schizophrenia can be treated with psychotherapy. My theory also
assumes the existence of endogenous biomedical subtypes of schizophrenia in which the principles of the trauma model do not apply and
for which trauma therapy is ineffective. The percentage of individuals
who belong to different subgroups is an empirical question—I have assumed, as argued earlier, that 25 to 40 percent of individuals in treatment for schizophrenia meet criteria for the dissociative subtype.

As in family systems theory, the presenting problem is actually a
solution to an unrecognized problem in the background. For instance,
self-mutilation usually serves the primary function of *mood-state
regulation*. The problem is intolerable feelings that last too long and
which are not dampened by the available repertoire of coping strategies. When the feelings are too bad for too long, it is time to self-
mutilate.

Self-mutilation is a highly effective technique of mood-state regulation, with an immediate onset of action. The bad feelings go away
instantly and are replaced by a warm, calm state of control and mastery. Similar to a heroin injection, however, the effect doesn't last
very long; the bad feelings return and the behavior is repeated. The
behavior is reinforced by the fact that it is very effective.

Similarly, people with bulimia would not purge after a binge episode if purging resulted in gaining twice as much weight. They purge
because it is a highly effective method for ridding the body of calo-
ries. All addictive behavior, I assume, is multifactorial in its causation. Many of the functions of binge and purge episodes, for instance,
may be unconscious. In cognitive therapy, the core beliefs and automatic negative thoughts are also regarded as "unconscious" in the
sense that they occur automatically without conscious awareness.
The purpose of cognitive therapy is first to identify them (make them
conscious), then to change them.

The first task facing the therapist is to understand the function of
the presenting problem, which is in fact a solution to some underlying
problem. The next task is to develop alternative, equally effective
coping strategies that are more healthy, fluid, and adaptive.

The idea that the problem is not the problem applies to auditory
hallucinations, Schneiderian passivity experiences, delusional thinking, and all other symptoms of psychosis within the trauma model.

Rector and Beck (2002) describe the application of therapy to hallucinations and delusions in schizophrenia. The purpose of the therapy, as they describe it, is not simply to assist with adjustment to medication-unresponsive residual symptoms but for direct remediation of psychotic symptoms. In addition, it can assist with indirect coping and general nonpsychotic cognitive errors, but it is an active treatment for the core symptoms of schizophrenia.

Within trauma therapy, I attempt to engage the voices in conversation. I explain to the person in treatment that I am going to ask the voices some questions. If they can, the voices will answer inside the person's head, and the person will tell me what they said. The voices may spontaneously assume executive control or may remain inside. Either way, the process provides a powerful experiential correction to core beliefs and cognitive errors. When the voices can engage in rational conversation, express a viewpoint, and participate in negotiations, the person learns that he or she is not "crazy." The voices become a disavowed and conflicted aspect of self, rather than alien intrusions caused by insanity or brain disease. I have provided a series of vignettes illustrating techniques and strategies for talking to the voices in *The Trauma Model* (Ross, 2000b).

Desensitization Is the Opposite of Addiction

The problem, in any addiction, is *here*. *Here* is intolerable feelings, conflicts, and life situations. The purpose of any addiction is to take you from *here* to *over there*. *Over there* is stoned, wasted, distracted, thrilled, passed out, or otherwise far away from the feelings and conflicts. All addictions, then, are avoidance strategies. Within the trauma model, anything can be an addiction—the patient role, trauma flashbacks, Internet sex, gambling, alcohol, command hallucinations, or the belief that one is the helpless victim of one's own defenses.

In the treatment of any addiction, the first step is to "just say no to drugs." The patient must make a serious, deep commitment to abstinence and sobriety. There is no procedure, manual, technique, or set of instructions for this task. It is a choice that no one else can make. Patients may trick other people into believing they are serious about recovery—they can even trick themselves—but in the long run, it won't work.

This principle is at the core of all twelve-step approaches to addictions, and I agree with it completely. The person must be accountable for all choices and decisions. The addiction may be experienced as overwhelming, involuntary, and irresistible, but it is not. Take self-mutilation, for instance.

Self-mutilation requires a long sequence of choices and decisions, all of them conscious, deliberate, functional, and goal directed. First, you have to acquire money. Then you have to save it and remember where it is. Next you have to check to make sure the money is in your purse or wallet. Then you have to get your car keys and walk to your car. If you were delirious or in the middle of a partial complex seizure, you might walk into the wall or be unable to turn the door handle. You have to put the keys in the ignition, and so on. You have to drive to a store that sells razor blades; a bakery won't work. You have to go to the shelf where the razor blades are, because you can't self-mutilate with shaving cream. You might check to see which razor blades are on sale. Then you pay for them, take them home, hide them, and decide not to tell your therapist or significant other about them. Then, one day, you are suddenly overcome with an irresistible urge to self-mutilate. You enter an altered state of consciousness and impulsively self-mutilate. You "just couldn't stop" yourself.

Perhaps you were even amnesic for the self-mutilation. But a long series of choices and decisions occurred before you spontaneously, impulsively cut yourself. Each one of these is a potential control point, an opportunity to make a different choice, and a chance to "say no to drugs."

By describing the chain of decisions in minute detail, I refute the proposition that the behavior is involuntary or irresistible. It is in fact carefully planned and serves a specific function, namely, avoidance of intolerable feelings, conflicts, and life situations.

Desensitization is the opposite of addiction. In desensitization, you turn around and face the thing you have been avoiding (which you do after having said no to drugs). There are two types of desensitization. At workshops I explain the first by saying that I dug a pit outside my hospital in Dallas and then put 300 snakes at the bottom.

Whenever someone with a snake phobia is admitted to my trauma program, I take him or her out for a walk and push the individual into the snake pit. Then I take a break for lunch. After lunch, I return to the snake pit, being careful not to get too close to the edge. I lean over the edge and call out to my patient, "Feeling better yet?"

This type of desensitization is called *flooding*. For survivors of complex trauma, flooding causes decompensation, melting down, regression, and an increase in symptoms and acting out. Therefore, within the trauma model, I recommend *systematic desensitization*.

In systematic desensitization, the therapist creates a structure, educates the patient about the vocabulary and rationale of treatment, constructs a desensitization hierarchy, and breaks the work down into the most minute microsteps necessary. For instance, I would first explain the logic and principles of systematic desensitization to my patient. I would then set them in the general context of the overall principles and goals of trauma therapy. This education itself provides a modicum of desensitization and begins to correct the cognitive error that the feelings are overwhelming, intolerable, and unmanageable.

I would teach and practice a set of grounding and distracting techniques. These could include simple behaviors by the patient such as standing up, shuffling his or her feet, looking around the office, or looking out the window. I might provide direct instructions to stop staring in one direction and I might say forcefully who I am, where we are, what the date is, and what is going on. I might remind the person that the traumatic events happened a long time ago, and I might point out that the person is now an adult, tall, strong, able to draw on healthy supports, and no longer living in the childhood home. All of these interventions help pull the person back into the present and away from blind abreaction.

The exposure component of the desensitization involves experiencing the phobic stimulus, which consists of disavowed feelings and conflicts. These can be evoked by telling the trauma narrative. Alternatively, I might ask the person to imagine what would happen if all addictions, all acting out, and all self-destructive coping strategies were instantly eliminated. Most likely the person would be flooded with feelings. Simply going through this hypothetically and asking what feelings would arise can evoke those feelings.

Desensitization has several purposes. Adult survivors of complex, chronic childhood traumas tend to be stuck in the past. They look at the world through the eyes of a traumatized, magical child. Their trauma-derived moods and feelings appear way too big, too intolerable, too engulfing, and too long lasting for anything but avoidance to make sense. In childhood, it was actually true that feeling or expressing emotions was dangerous—it would often provoke neglect or retaliation by caretakers. Now, thirty years later, the person is still living by the rule that feelings are too dangerous to be felt.

The purpose of desensitization, then, is to provide a safe, contained, structured forum in which to reexperience the feelings and correct the cognitive error. The person must be grounded and have rational adult faculties intact. When the feelings are reexperienced in a grounded, adult mental state, the person learns that they are not as huge and unmanageable as predicted. This results in desensitization.

In the next session the person can go further into the feelings, having learned that it is possible to de-escalate and back out of them without unhealthy or addictive behaviors. The phobic stimulus, in this model, is primarily a set of internal feelings, mood states, and memories. The principles of desensitization, however, are the same as those for behavioral therapy of a single external phobia such as blood, needles, or specific animals. Simply talking about and feeling the feelings without acting out results in desensitization.

Patients often ask what they should do with the feelings if they don't act out in order to avoid them. The fundamental answer is, nothing. The goal is to feel the feelings, not do anything with them. Doing so in a grounded, adult state results in desensitization and reduces the likelihood of catastrophy. The feelings appear less overwhelming and it becomes more plausible that they can be coped with using healthy defenses. The realistic optimism engendered by the model leads to a self-fulfilling prophecy—the belief that the feelings are intolerable changes and they in fact become tolerable. This requires practice and is an arduous and painful process, but the model sets up a realistic hope for recovery, which provides motivation to do the work. Much of this is achieved through education.

The second function of the work is to build affect management skills. However, an arid, intellectualized, didactic format has limited usefulness. In structured experiential groups in my trauma programs, we carry out exercises to get the feelings up and running. Because the feelings are intensely present, it is no longer a merely intellectual exercise. The person has to practice healthy containment and self-soothing in an aroused state that closely approximates the real world.

Because the experiential exercise is more similar to an in vivo than an in vitro exposure technique, it is more generalizable.

The process is reciprocal. Patients learn healthier affect management skills by practicing them. The practice makes the affect more manageable. To practice, however, the affect must first be present. Also, patients must first learn skills that make the practice safe. The two processes go on in a simultaneous and alternating fashion. It is not a simple linear sequence of activities.

Generally, patients enter therapy with a pattern of experiencing too much affect, which is then suppressed through self-mutilation, substance abuse, bulimia, or other behaviors. The affect is then absent until it suddenly intrudes in a forceful, overwhelming manner, only to be suppressed again with addictive behaviors. These are the two poles of numbing and hyperarousal that are incorporated in the DSM-IV-TR criteria for PTSD.

Desensitization, then, has two equally important elements: going into the feelings and backing out of them without resorting to unhealthy defenses or behaviors. The third, and minor, function of the work is *catharsis*. It is helpful to blow off steam or have a good cry. The staff educates the patients in my trauma programs about the rationale and vocabulary of desensitization just as a behavioral therapist would do in an office or laboratory setting. Desensitization is taught and practiced in both individual and group psychotherapy formats in the trauma programs.

Once desensitization has occurred and healthy cognitions and coping strategies have been learned and practiced, the need for the addictions melts away. There is then no need to solve the presenting problem because the underlying problem has been solved. The addictions and unhealthy defenses are no longer required because they are redundant and have been replaced. Desensitization and affect management skill building make it possible to construct a trauma narrative without malignant abreaction or regression.

The Problem of Attachment to the Perpetrator

The basic assumption of the treatment model is that organisms want to survive. For most species, this involves taking off into the swamp or jungle immediately after birth, sometimes to evade the jaws of the biological parents. For mammals and birds, however, survival depends absolutely on the presence of an adult caretaker.

Built into birds and mammals is a complex set of attachment mechanisms, which are reciprocal between parents and child. This is similar to the migration of birds or a chameleon changing colors—it is not done by choice or conscious decision; rather it is biology. A mammal will, must, and does attach.

In an average, reasonably healthy family a child is faced with the problem of attachment to the "perpetrator." The parent perpetrates on the child the "crime" of being imperfectly attuned, attentive, and protective. The outcome of this developmental process is what I call an *average neurotic mess*. We all have a love-hate, on-off, approach-avoidance conflict with our parents. This is just the human condition, even when the family is healthy, and the word *perpetrator* is used to describe the parents only as an analogy.

However, some children experience the problem of attachment to the perpetrator to an extreme degree. They come from trauma families characterized by severe, chronic abuse, neglect, violence, and chaos. As adults they arrive at my trauma program with split, ambivalent attachment patterns dominating their relationships in the present. They exhibit the "I hate you; don't leave me" approach-avoidance conflicts that are at the core of borderline personality disorder. In the DSM-IV-TR these appear as the diagnostic criterion for idealization and devaluation.

Highly conflicted, ambivalent, and dichotomized attachment patterns are a logical, predictable outcome of the problem of attachment to the perpetrator. A child in a major trauma family is trying to do two things simultaneously or in a chaotic sequence: attach and flee; approach and avoid; love and hate. The child wants to be special in the eyes of the caretaker, and be loved and protected by the caretaker, and simultaneously fears and recoils from the caretaker, who is the most dangerous person in his or her world.

The assumption of the model is that the imperative to attach overrides the instinct to flee. The basic goal is survival. To survive, one must attach. To attach, Mom and Dad must be safe to attach to. For this to be true, the bad stuff must be put aside.

This basic need to protect the attachment systems drives the fundamental splitting, dissociation, fracturing, or fragmenting of the internal world. In ego psychology terms, the result is a set of ambivalently held part-object identifications. In cognitive therapy terms, there is a basic dichotomization, personalization, catatrophization, and over-generalization. I derived the role of attachment in the trauma model from two sources: my patients and Jennifer Freyd's (1996) betrayal trauma theory. She taught me that the fundamental role of trauma-driven dissociation is not to protect feelings but to maintain attachment. Jennifer Freyd's book helped me return to earlier articles on trauma, dissociation, and attachment (Barach, 1991; Liotti, 1992) and appreciate their significance more clearly.

According to both betrayal trauma theory and the trauma model, in childhood the abusive parent and the safe parent cannot be simultaneously present, because that would threaten the security of attachment. The bad parent has to be banished, from the perspective of the attachment systems. This is done through dissociation, which maintains an illusion that the parents are safe attachment figures. Disconfirming experience and evidence are held in dissociated compartments of the psyche. The reverse is also true. Dissociation allows the child, from one dissociated perspective, to experience the parent as purely bad without any intrusion of disconfirming positive data and experience.

In adulthood, this pattern persists because it is still too painful to feel both halves of the dichotomized, conflicted attachment. If the patient is currently a battered wife whose husband might kill her if she leaves, the childhood dependency on an adult caretaker for biological survival has been replicated. The current marriage is a reenactment of the relationship between the enraged, alcoholic father and the child.

The work of therapy, then, is integration. The basic fact that must be accepted, first in the head and then in the heart, is *I loved the people who hurt me, and I was hurt by the people I loved.* It is feeling both these feelings at the same time that is intolerable. A person can hide in one feeling to avoid the other, oscillate back and forth from one to the other in an endless borderline dance, or avoid the whole mess through addictions. But once a person makes a commitment to recovery and begins the work of desensitization, then the basic truth begins to set in.

This realization throws clients into the fundamental work of recovery, which is mourning the loss of the parents they never actually had.

The parents they never had were halfway reasonable, consistent, safe parents who were there for them most of the time. Instead, the parents they actually grew up with provided a chaotic, threatening mixture of affection, abuse, and neglect. Recovery, within this model, is basically a process of mourning, loss, and grief resolution. The underlying feeling that is being avoided is that of a small, scared, lost, lonely, and sad child. People pay very high costs to avoid this underlying reality.

One feature of the model is that recovery is not primarily about specific bad events that took place. At the deepest level, the trauma is not event specific; rather it is about the entire gestalt of childhood: "my parents just weren't there for me." Thus the fundamental work of therapy cannot involve processing memories of specific events, and cannot be focused on memory content. It is more about the errors of omission by the parents than the errors of commission. It is about the good things they didn't do more than the bad things they did do.

This doesn't mean that there is no processing of events that meet Criterion A, the trauma criterion for PTSD. The work still involves construction of a trauma narrative, but a deeper layer of grief drives the defenses, acting out, symptoms, diagnoses, and addictions. It is a matter of a balance between the deeper grief work and the construction of an event-specific trauma narrative.

The Locus of Control Shift

The scientific foundation of the locus of control shift is Piaget and developmental psychology; for the problem of attachment to the perpetrator, it is the biology of mammalian attachment. Developmental psychology tells us what we already know from common sense and common experience: kids think like kids. The young child is at the center of his or her own world; the world revolves around him or her; he or she causes everything that happens in his or her world; and he or she has a magical power to make things happen. Of course, the literature on developmental psychology, including Piaget, is rich, complex, and far more intricate than this simple summary.

The mind of the magical child is alive and well, dominating life in the present thirty years later when the adult survivor is admitted to my trauma program. In psychoanalytical terms, there has been a developmental fixation—in cognitive therapy terms, there are persisting maladaptive core beliefs and cognitive errors.

Consider a four-year-old girl in a relatively normal family. Everything is okay until a very sad day in her life: her parents split up and her dad moves out. What is true for this little girl? She is overwhelmed, powerless, helpless, trapped in her situation, sad, and lonely. She feels the feelings that match her reality.

Then she shifts the locus of control. This occurs automatically because of her developmentally normal cognition. The little girl says to herself, "I know why Daddy doesn't live here anymore. It's because I didn't keep my bedroom tidy."

This is not true. It is a cognitive error. But it is the inevitable outcome of the operations of a normal four-year-old mind. The locus of control shift is not driven by gender, race, culture, personal feelings, or peculiarities of the individual. It happens because all children think this way. Children shift power, control, and mastery over the situation from inside the adults in their world to inside themselves.

The price of this shift is badness of the self. "I am bad; I caused Daddy to leave me." But there is also a benefit. Once she realizes that her father moved out because of her messy bedroom, the little girl is no longer powerless, helpless, or lost without a future. The problem is contained within herself; and she has a solution. All she has to do is tidy up her bedroom, and Daddy will move back home. Now she is able to form other attachments and carry out her developmental tasks because she is buffered from the full impact of her trauma. The world is okay, or at least, it will be okay soon.

The locus of control shift provides a developmentally protective illusion of power, control, and mastery at the cost of the badness of the self. Imagine a child in a major trauma family. When this child is admitted to my trauma program thirty years later, the locus of control shift is still in place and still dominating her thoughts, feelings, and behavior in the present.

In my experience, survivors of serious, chronic childhood trauma who are early in their recovery, who meet criteria for numerous DSM-IV-TR disorders, and who have multiple addictions and self-defeating behaviors almost always endorse the locus of control shift. They state aloud that they are bad, that they caused their abuse, and that they deserved it. They know this to be true about themselves with absolute certainty. Child abuse breeds self-hatred.

At the same time, most people in my trauma programs will state that no one else in the program, and no other child in the history of the human race, caused or deserved his or her abuse. Why does this cognitive error persist? Because it provides an illusion of power and control.

The locus of control shift has one unfortunate property—it is prone to decay or spontaneous reversal, in response to accumulated positive experiences in life. A person might learn that he or she is not bad and did not cause the childhood misery. This would be a bad thing for several reasons. First, letting go of badness of the self will destroy the illusion of power, control, and mastery, exposing the person to the underlying feelings of the scared, lost, lonely child.

By taking all the causality and all the badness inside the self, the child made the parents be all good. This made them safe attachment figures and solved the problem of attachment to the perpetrator.

When the locus of control shift is reversed in adulthood, a question arises: "If I was not bad, then who was?" The answer is not far to seek: "My parents." Reversal of the shift shatters the illusion of the bad self, but then brings the person face to face with reality: I loved the people who hurt me, and I was hurt by the people I loved. Now, both poles of the split, ambivalent feelings, are felt at the same time. This throws people into the fundamental work of recovery—mourning the loss of the parents they never actually had.

The locus of control shift, then, is a major strategy of grief avoidance. Since it might decay or reverse itself in response to positive experience, it must be reinforced. This is done through negative self-talk, negative, unhealthy behavior directed at the self, and by contracting with outside people to treat you badly in word and deed. Case in point: the battered wife who goes back to her husband, vowing to improve her performance so that the abuse will stop.

Negative auditory and command hallucinations are a depersonalized variant of old thoughts. They reinforce belief in the bad self, and provide examples of a basic therapeutic principle: the problem is not the problem. The problem is the grief and, as in all addictions, intolerable feelings, conflicts, and life situations. It is good to have voices telling you that you are bad, because then you can hold onto the illusion of power, control, and mastery. Everything will be okay if you punish the self one more time, or if an outside person explains to you that the self is bad, diseased, insane, or a genetic mutant.

Engaging negative voices in therapy should be attempted only when the patient is sufficiently stable. Basic safety, trust, and a treatment alliance must be in place. The individual must understand the principles, rules, and goals of therapy and must be able to tolerate unpleasant feelings, limit acting out, and delay gratification like anyone who participates in psychotherapy. Given these prerequisites, voices are more likely to engage in therapy when they are articulate, interactive with other voices or the executive self, and intellectually organized. Voices that are rigid, fixed, unintelligible, or infrequent are less likely to be engaged.

The clinician should imagine that there is another "person" inside. The decision to interview this other person therapeutically should be based on the same principles as interviewing in general. If the body in which this person lives is violent, highly agitated, or threatening, an attempt at psychotherapy is more likely to be delayed. If the person mutters unintelligibly, this is not a good prognostic sign, and so on.

The first step in reversing the locus of control shift is education about it. The second is cognitive therapy designed to reject the false belief at an intellectual level. The third is letting go of the badness of the self at the level of core belief—"in your heart." To do this work, one must reject self-hatred, set up a desensitization hierarchy, and do the grief work that will eventually make the cognitive errors, addictions, auditory hallucinations, and self-defeating behaviors superfluous.

There is more to grieve than just a lost childhood. There are also the lost hopes, dreams, and opportunities of adulthood and the wake of misery due to years of addiction and acting out. The basic twelve-step tasks of making a fearless inventory and making amends bring with them a lot of grief and mourning. It is painful and difficult work, but it is the only road I know out of the swamp of despair, psychosis, and addiction.

As I shift from scholarly argument and analysis of data to therapy, my language becomes more simple and nontechnical, except for a few basic terms and ideas. The trauma model is designed so that it can be learned, remembered, and used by both therapist and patient. It includes only a few basic ideas. A more detailed explication is available in Ross (1989, 1994, 1995, 1997, 2000b).

The purpose of this book is not to train mental health professionals in trauma therapy. There must be a sequence of steps. First, the theory of a dissociative subtype of schizophrenia must be accepted. That is, a number of clinicians, scholars, and researchers must agree that it is worth investing serious time, energy, and resources in study of dissociative schizophrenia.

If this occurs, more data will be required on the phenomenology, reliability, and validity of the diagnostic category. Only then will it make sense to fund and carry out a series of rigorous psychotherapy outcome studies. These will require both a manual version of the therapy and a book devoted solely to principles, strategies, and techniques. Here I have attempted to give the reader a basic sense of what the therapy entails.

Chapter 17

Talking to the Voices

The single most revolutionary principle of the psychotherapy of dissociative schizophrenia is talking to the voices. This is simply not done in contemporary psychiatry. The model of schizophrenia does not allow it. Within contemporary biological psychiatry, the symptoms of schizophrenia have no psychological meaning or purpose. There is no need to perform a microdetailed mental status examination because the findings have no influence on diagnosis, the theory of etiology, treatment planning, or the design of research protocols.

Attention to psychopathological detail such as we see in Bleuler (1950 [1911]) has become superfluous in contemporary psychiatry, similar to the numerous ways of cataloging and describing the pulse in nineteenth-century medicine. These were abandoned because they had no specific effect on treatment planning, and because they were supplanted by echocardiograms, angiograms, X rays, enzyme blood levels, and other modern technologies. Similarly, in contemporary biological psychiatry, once auditory hallucinations are documented, there is no need to find out details about them; the treatment plan is antipsychotic medication and the choice of neuroleptic is not affected by the features of the voices.

There is another, more fundamental reason not to talk to the voices in contemporary psychiatry: the voices are not the patient. The patient is the patient; the voices are a symptom with which the patient is afflicted. The doctor tries to form a treatment alliance with the patient to foster compliance with the treatment plan, which is to rid the patient of symptoms. When the symptoms are gone, the patient is better, or at least improved.

Voices, then, are similar to swelling and pain in a joint. The doctor prescribes a medication to relieve inflammation in the joint; it would never occur to him or her to ask the inflammation a question. If the doctor did, he or she would be an impaired physician. This medical relationship between doctor, patient, and symptoms has been copied by psychiatry.

Within the trauma model, however, the voices have psychological meaning, function, and purpose. The doctor must understand the meaning of the symptoms in order to plan treatment. The paradigm shift has another, more fundamental element, however. *Paradigm shift* is a term coined by Thomas Kuhn (1962) to describe discontinuous shifts in the advancement of science. The classical example is the shift from Newtonian physics to relativity theory and quantum mechanics.

Prior to a paradigm shift, a given field of science is dominated by an accepted model. Research within the model, called *normal science* by Kuhn, does not challenge or question the model's basic rules and assumptions. Gradually, however, anomalous observations accumulate until they reach a critical mass. These observations cannot be accounted for by the dominant model and are ignored or discredited by its adherents.

What happens next is a paradigm shift to a new model and a new way of seeing things. The old model is a subset of the new one—the new model can account for all the phenomena explained by its predecessor but also makes sense of the anomalous data. It leads to new studies, observations, and predictions that could not arise from the old model. In physics, Einsteinian equations can be used to solve all problems dealt with by Newtonian equations; Einstein's equations yield the same answers as Newton's when acceleration is set at zero. In accelerating systems, however, Einstein's equations can account for observations and make accurate predictions that are not possible using Newtonian equations.

Similarly, the theory of a dissociative subtype of schizophrenia leads to observations, predictions, research projects, and clinical interventions that could not arise from conventional psychiatry. Within conventional psychiatry, talking to the voices makes no sense. However, the responses of the voices to questioning by a psychiatrist can lead to differential treatment planning within my theory.

In my worldview, the voices are also the patient. They are not products of biological defect and error. Nor are they simply "defenses." They are dissociated elements of the person. They are as much the person as the person, despite the patient's denial of that fact. My goal here is to clarify the rationale for talking to the voices, not to explain the techniques for doing so in any detail.

Briefly, however, I talk to the voices as if they are other people living inside the person's head. I ask them if they can hear me, if they have anything to say, and specifically if they have any comments on the session to date. Then I may proceed with more specific questions. For instance, I might ask, "If Tom would agree to stop watching horror movies on TV, would you agree to stop screaming at him?"

This question would be based on Tom's report that when he watches horror movies, one of the voices becomes agitated and angry and threatens him with death. The more the voice can be engaged in a therapeutic conversation, the more likely it is that Tom has the dissociative subtype of schizophrenia. If the voices are more fixed and invariable, do not respond to probes from the psychiatrist, and make only a limited number of stereotyped statements, it is less likely that the person has dissociative schizophrenia.

I want to form a treatment alliance with the voices, understand their point of view, and engage them in the therapy process. One of my goals is to create more empathy for them in the patient. Eventually, I want to integrate the dissociated thoughts, feelings, and perceptions of the voices into a whole identity. When the voices become part of the person, the person no longer experiences auditory hallucinations or Schneiderian intrusions by dissociated part-selves.

The psychotic symptoms follow logically from the dissociated part-self structure of the psyche. They are not the problem; rather, they are a logical outcome of a fragmented, conflicted psyche that disavows ownership of its own impulses, thoughts, feelings, and conflicts. When the person with dissociative schizophrenia asks me to suppress his or her command hallucinations to self-mutilate, I certainly want to prevent the behavior from occurring, but I don't want to get rid of the voices. They are commanding self-harm to protect the patient from feelings and conflicts. They are defenses, not symptoms of biological brain disease.

Defining the voices as meaningless products of malfunctioning brain circuitry is helpful if the goal is to reinforce denial, dissociation, internal conflict, and fragmentation. For some people, this may be the only realistic treatment goal. A person with schizophrenia may lack the motivation, resources, social support, physical health, or other motivators and requirements for the hard work of psychotherapy. For such people, conventional treatment is all psychiatry has to offer. If a person has an endogenous disease form of schizophrenia, psychotherapy for the psychosis might be of less use or no use at all. In this scenario, however, psychotherapy could still be of benefit for general coping and for adjustment to the disease.

For people with the dissociative subtype of schizophrenia, the current biomedical model provides the patient with a rationalization for suppression of disavowed aspects of the self. It interferes with treatment and recovery. Unfortunately, as I know from efficacy data on neuroleptic medication, the promise to suppress the voices with medication is usually not realistic. Seventy percent of schizophrenic persons prescribed antipsychotic medications are nonresponders, according to data submitted to the Food and Drug Administration and published in professional journals. Suppressing the voices with medication doesn't work for most people.

The trauma model of dissociative schizophrenia is medical, scientific, scholarly, scientifically testable, operationalized, and microdetailed. It is based on an alternative scientific model of the brain-mind field. The theory is not proven, but that is not a criticism of it. The purpose of the theory is to stimulate the gathering of new data. If the data already existed and were incorporated into conventional psychiatry, there would be no need for the theory or this book.

Within bioreductionist psychiatry, causality for schizophrenia and other severe forms of mental disorder runs in only one direction: from soma to psyche. Once the disorder in the soma is fully understood, at some point in the future, definitive treatment will be purely physical, according to the bioreductionist model. The psychosocial realm is merely a trigger; at most it can modify the content of symptoms or hasten the onset of a psychotic episode. The psychosocial environment is alluded to in brief comments about "stress" within contemporary biological psychiatry but is not otherwise investigated, and there are no specific treatment techniques for it other than simple stress reduction and social work interventions.

Within the trauma model, causality for severe mental disorders can run in both directions: from soma to psyche, and from psyche to soma. I predict that there are numerous interacting feedback loops running in both directions. The trauma model assumes that psychological trauma causes measurable damage to the central nervous system. The structures, neurotransmitters, and functions affected can be specified, demonstrated in animal models, and targeted in treatment.

For example, excess excitatory glutaminergic neurotransmission in the hippocampus combined with high levels of circulating cortisol, both caused by psychological trauma, could cause hippocampal damage, which could produce a failure to integrate the components of thought, feeling, identity, arousal, and perception. This failure of integration could be simultaneously a biological effect of trauma and a psychological defense against trauma—the hippocampal damage could facilitate dissociation, which in turn could serve a psychological function. It is conceivable that, once in place, the dissociation could cause further deterioration of circuits designed to integrate thought, feeling, identity, arousal, and perception through disuse atrophy. The bioreductionist model is wrong because it is too simple.

I further predict that a traumatized individual can repair the biological damage caused by the genetically normal trauma response through psychotherapy; in the therapy of DID, techniques to enhance communication, cooperation, and integration of function among alter personalities also train damaged hippocampal neurons to communicate effectively in a subtle, functional, psychologically meaningful fashion. The psychotherapy teaches the neuronal circuits how to integrate. To reiterate, these statements are predictions, not facts. I make them to illustrate how the theory leads to specific research predictions that could not arise from bioreductionist psychiatry.

According to my theory, trauma therapy stimulates neuronal self-repair and also organizes it in a functional manner that enhances adaptation to the psychosocial environment. The regeneration of dendritic connections between hippocampal neurons is structured and psychologically rational. The mind tells the brain how to rewire itself.

This property of the brain-mind field is not allowed by the bioreductionist model. The difference between the two models is basic; the physics of the brain-mind field differ in the two paradigms. Within my model, the decision to engage the voices in a therapeutic conversation initiates a cascade of electromagnetic reorganization in the brain-mind field that is detectable on EEG, assuming a sensitive enough gauge.

Through a trickle-down effect, the electromagnetic changes alter the environment of ions, gates, and molecules in the central nervous system. These then activate genes, neurotrophic factors, neuronal transport mechanisms, and a wide range of biological machinery. The outcome of this process is organized dendritic growth; SSRI medications can provide a structurally nonspecific stimulus to regeneration but cannot provide the organizational guidance necessary to carry out simultaneous biological and functional repair.

Talking to the voices provides the brain with a model of how to talk to itself. It is the brain self-talk that is healing.

Although we lack technology of sufficient precision to make all the relevant measurements to prove or disprove my model, we can test it with currently available treatment outcome designs, psychometrics, brain scans, and blood tests. These can be combined with a variety of chemical and neuropsychological challenges and tasks. The brain is not a machine because it possesses properties absent in Newtonian machines; it can initiate and carry out self-repair through verbal language.

The self-destructive biological feedback loops activated by psychological trauma are not derived from diagnostically specific abnormalities in the genome, within my model. The negative effects of high cortisol levels on hippocampal neurons are not caused by a gene or genes for a specific psychiatric disorder. They are caused by the response of the normal genome and soma to this form of toxic environmental input. There is no abnormal gene to find, only normal genes that were not designed to solve an environmental problem; if these normal genes are never selected against, they will never disappear from the gene pool.

Given the short average life span of human beings up till a few hundred years ago, and the low average age of pregnant women, there was little or no opportunity for adult PTSD, dissociative disorders, or dissociative schizophrenia to be selected against through reduced fertility. This may still be the case—another prediction of the model is higher fertility rates among individuals with dissociative schizophrenia than among those with other subtypes. Individuals with dissociative schizophrenia have fewer negative and more positive symptoms; therefore they may have more success in attracting sexual partners. In some cultures, the positive symptoms may be prized as evidence of shamanic talent, divine calling, or spiritual power; therefore they may confer a survival advantage. This is a specific, testable prediction of the model that could not arise from bioreductionist psychiatry.

In closing, I thank my patients and my colleagues for the lessons they have taught me concerning trauma, dissociation, and psychosis. I ask the mental health field to consider and weigh my data, arguments, and model in a dispassionate and rational manner. The theory of a dissociative subtype of schizophrenia is based on the collective work of many people. The theory was not possible when Bleuler wrote his 1911 text on dementia praecox. In 1911, there was no reliable system of diagnosis, no structured diagnostic interviews, and no valid and reliable measures of pathological dissociation. No model of psychotherapy existed that allowed the therapist to talk to the voices, and there was no field of trauma studies.

In 1911 the culture was not receptive to a trauma model of mental disorders and addictions. Freud repudiated the seduction theory late in the nineteenth century (Masson, 1985), and the culture followed his lead. Now things are different. Childhood trauma and its consequences are widely recognized. A large body of data supports a trauma model of psychosis. None of these elements existed for Bleuler; therefore he could not fit his observations into a scientifically testable model. The theory of a dissociative subtype of schizophrenia pays homage to Bleuler and builds on the clinical work he did a century ago.

Bibliography

Agar, K., and Read, J. (2002). What happens when people disclose sexual or physical abuse to staff at a community mental health center? *International Journal of Mental Health Nursing,* 11, 7-79.

Akyuz, G., Dogan, O., Sar, V., Yargic, L.I., and Tutkun, H. (1999). Frequency of dissociative identity disorder in the general population in Turkey. *Comprehensive Psychiatry,* 40, 151-159.

Allen, J.G. (2001). *Traumatic relationships and serious mental disorders.* New York: John Wiley and Sons.

Allen, J.G., Coyne, L., and Console, D.A. (1996). Dissociation contributes to anxiety and psychoticism on the Brief Symptom Inventory. *Journal of Nervous and Mental Disease,* 184, 639-641.

Ambelas, A. (1992). Preschizophrenics: Adding to the evidence, sharpening the focus. *British Journal of Psychiatry,* 160, 401-444.

American Psychiatric Association (1980). *Diagnostic and statistical manual of mental disorders* (Third edition). Washington, DC: American Psychiatric Association.

American Psychiatric Association (1987). *Diagnostic and statistical manual of mental disorders* (Third edition, revised). Washington, DC: American Psychiatric Association.

American Psychiatric Association (1994). *Diagnostic and statistical manual of mental disorders* (Fourth edition). Washington, DC: American Psychiatric Association.

American Psychiatric Association (2000). *Diagnostic and statistical manual of mental disorders* (Fourth edition, text revision). Washington, DC: American Psychiatric Association.

Andreasen, N.C. (1983). *Scale for the Assessment of Negative Symptoms (SANS).* Iowa City: University of Iowa.

Andreasen, N.C. (1984). *Scale for the Assessment of Positive Symptoms (SAPS).* Iowa City: University of Iowa.

Armstrong, J. (1991). The psychological organization of multiple personality disordered patients as revealed in psychological testing. *Psychiatric Clinics of North America,* 14, 533-548.

Armstrong, J.G., and Loewenstein, R.G. (1990). Characteristics of patients with multiple personality and dissociative disorders on psychological testing. *Journal of Nervous and Mental Disease,* 178, 448-464.

Arvantis, L.A., and Miller, B.G. (1997). Multiple fixed doses of "Seroquel" (quetiapine) in patients with acute exacerbations of schizophrenia: A comparison with haloperidol and placebo. *Biological Psychiatry,* 42, 233-246.

Bachmann, S., Resch, F., and Mundt, C. (2003). Psychological treatments for psychosis: History and overview. *Journal of the American Academy of Psychoanalysis and Dynamic Psychiatry*, 31, 155-176.

Barach, P.M.M. (1991). Multiple personality disorder as an attachment disorder. *Dissociation*, 4, 117-123.

Barker-Collo, S. (2001). Adult reports of child and attributions of blame for childhood sexual abuse. Predicting adult adjustment and suicidal behaviors in females. *Child Abuse and Neglect*, 25, 1329-1341.

Barton, C. (1994a). Backstage in psychiatry: The multiple personality disorder controversy. *Dissociation*, 7, 167-172.

Barton, C. (1994b). More from backstage: A rejoinder to Merskey. *Dissociation*, 7, 176-177.

Beardslee, W.R., and Vaillant, G. (1997). Adult development. In A. Tasman, J. Kay, and J.A. Lieberman (Eds.), *Psychiatry* (pp. 145-155). Philadelphia: W.B. Saunders.

Bebbington, P., Wilkins, S., Jones, P., Foerster, A., Murray, R., Toone, B., and Lewis, S. (1993). Life events and psychosis. Initial results from the Camberwell collaborative psychosis study. *British Journal of Psychiatry*, 162, 72-79.

Beck, A.T., and Emery, G. (1985). *Anxiety disorders and phobias: A cognitive perspective*. New York: Basic Books.

Beck, A.T., Rush, A.J., Shaw, B.F., and Emery, G. (1979). *Cognitive therapy of depression*. New York: The Guilford Press.

Beck, J., and van der Kolk, B. (1987). Reports of childhood incest and current behavior of chronically hospitalized psychotic women. *American Journal of Psychiatry*, 144, 1474-1176.

Beitchman, J., Zucker, K., Hood, J., Dacosta, G., Ackman, D., and Cassavia, E. (1992). A review of the long-term effects of child sexual abuse. *Child Abuse and Neglect*, 16, 101-118.

Bentall, R. (1990). *Reconstructing schizophrenia*. New York: Routledge.

Bentall, R., and Kaney, S. (1996). Abnormalities of self-representation and persecutory delusions: A test of a cognitive model of paranoia. *Psychological Medicine*, 26, 1231-1237.

Bercel, N.A. (1959). A study of the influence of schizophrenic serum on the behavior of the spider: Zilla-x-notata. In D.D. Jackson (Ed.), *The etiology of schizophrenia* (pp. 159-174). New York: Basic Books.

Berenbaum, H. (1999). Peculiarity and reported child maltreatment. *Psychiatry*, 62, 21-35.

Berger, D., Sato, S., Ono, Y., Tezuka, I., Shirahase, J., Kuboki, T., and Suematsu, H. (1994). Dissociation and child abuse histories in an eating disorder cohort in Japan. *Acta Psychiatrica Scandinavia*, 90, 274-280.

Bernat, J.A., Ronfeldt, H.M., Calhoun, K.S., and Arias, I. (1998). Prevalence of traumatic events and peritraumatic predictors of posttraumatic stress symptoms in a nonclinical sample of college students. *Journal of Traumatic Stress*, 11, 645-664.

Bernstein, E.M., and Putnam, F.W. (1986). Development, reliability, and validity of a dissociation scale. *Journal of Nervous and Mental Disease*, 174, 727-735.

Bernstein, I., Ellason, J.W., Ross, C.A., and Vanerlinden, J. (2001). On the dimensionalities of the Dissociative Experiences Scale (DES) and the Dissociation Questionnaire (DIS-Q). *Journal of Trauma and Dissociation,* 2, 103-123.

Blazer, D.G., Kessler, R.C., McGonagle, K.A., and Swartz, M.S. (1994). The prevalence and distribution of major depression in a national community sample: The National Comorbidity Survey. *American Journal of Psychiatry,* 151, 979-986.

Bleuler, E. (1950 [1911]). *Dementia praecox or the group of schizophrenias.* New York: International Universities Press.

Bliss, E.L. (1980). Multiple personalities: A report of 14 cases with implications for schizophrenia. *Archives of General Psychiatry,* 37, 1388-1397.

Bola, J.R., and Mosher, L.R. (2003). Treatment of acute psychosis without neuroleptics: Two-year outcomes from the Soteria Project. *Journal of Nervous and Mental Disease,* 191, 219-229.

Boney-McCoy, S., and Finkelhor, D. (1995). Psychosocial sequelae of violent victimization in a national youth sample. *Journal of Consulting and Clinical Psychology,* 63, 726-736.

Boon, S., and Draijer, N. (1993). *Multiple personality disorder in the Netherlands.* Amsterdam: Swets & Zeitlinger.

Boyle, M. (1990). *Schizophrenia: A scientific delusion?* New York: Routledge.

Braude, S.E. (1995). *First-person plural: Multiple personality and the philosophy of mind* (Revised edition). London: Rowman and Littlefield.

Braun, B.G. (1986). *Treatment of multiple personality disorder.* Washington, DC: American Psychiatric Press.

Bremner, J.D. (2002). *Does stress damage the brain?* New York: W.W. Norton.

Bremner, J.D., and Brett, E. (1997). Trauma-related dissociative states and long-term psychopathology in posttraumatic stress disorder. *Journal of Traumatic Stress,* 10, 37-49.

Bremner, J.D., Krystal, J.H., Putnam, F.W., Southwick, S.M., Marmar, C., Charney, D.S., and Mazure, C.M. (1998). Measurement of dissociative states with the Clinician-Administered Dissociative States Scale (CADSS). *Journal of Traumatic Stress,* 11, 125-136.

Bremner, J.D., Krystal, J.H., Southwick, S.M., and Charney, D.S. (1995). Functional neuroanatomical correlates of the effects of stress on memory. *Journal of Traumatic Stress,* 4, 527-553.

Bremner, J.D., and Marmar, C.R. (1998). *Trauma, memory, and dissociation.* Washington, DC: American Psychiatric Press.

Bremner, J.D., Vermetten, E., Southwick, S.M., Krystal, J.H., and Charney, D.S. (1998). Trauma, memory, and dissociation: An integrative formulation. In J.D. Bremner and C.R. Marmar (Eds.), *Trauma, memory, and dissociation* (pp. 365-402). Washington, DC: American Psychiatric Press.

Brenner, I. (2001). *Dissociation of trauma: Theory, phenomenology, and technique.* Madison, CT: International Universities Press.

Breuer, J., and Freud, S. (1986 [1895]). *Studies on hysteria.* New York: Pelican Books.

Briere, J., and Conte, J. (1993). Self-reported amnesia for abuse in adults molested as children. *Journal of Traumatic Stress,* 6, 21-31.

Briere, J., Woo, R., McRae, B., Foltz, J., and Sitzman, R. (1997). Lifetime victimization history, demographics, and clinical status in female psychiatric emergency room patients. *Journal of Nervous and Mental Disease,* 185, 95-101.

Brodsky, B.S., Oquendo, M., Ellis, S.P., Haas, G.L., Malone, K.M., and Mann, J.J. (2001). The relationship of childhood abuse to impulsivity and suicidal behavior in adults with major depression. *American Journal of Psychiatry,* 158, 1871-1877.

Brown, D. (2002). (Mis)representations of the long-term effects of childhood sexual abuse in the courts. *Journal of Child Sexual Abuse,* 9, 79-108.

Brown, D., and Scheflin, A.W. (1999). Editor's page. *Journal of Psychiatry and the Law,* 27, 367-372.

Brown, D., Scheflin, A.W., and Hammond, D.C. (1998). *Memory, trauma treatment, and the law.* New York: W.W. Norton.

Brown, D., Scheflin, A.W., and Whitfield, C.L. (1999). Recovered memories: The current weight of the evidence in science and the courts. *Journal of Psychiatry and the Law,* 27, 5-156.

Bryer, J., Nelson, B., Miller, J., and Krol, P. (1987). Childhood sexual and physical abuse as factors in psychiatric illness. *American Journal of Psychiatry,* 144, 1426-1430.

Bustillo, J.R., Laurillo, J., Horan, W.P., and Keith, S.J. (2001). The psychosocial treatment of schizophrenia: An update. *American Journal of Psychiatry,* 158, 163-175.

Butler, R.W., Mueser, K.T., Sprock, J., and Braff, D.L. (1996). Positive symptoms of psychosis in posttraumatic stress disorder. *Biological Psychiatry,* 39, 839-844.

Cairns, S. (1998). MMPI-2 and Rorschach assessments of adults physically abused as children. Unpublished doctoral dissertation, University of Manitoba.

Cannon, M., Walsh, E., Hollis, C., Maresc, K., Taylor, E., Murray, R., and Jones, P. (2001). Predictors of later schizophrenia and affective psychoses among attendees at a child psychiatry department. *British Journal of Psychiatry,* 178, 420-426.

Cannon, T.D., Kaprio, J., Lonnqvist, J., Huttunen, M., and Koskenvuo, M. (1998). The genetic epidemiology of schizophrenia in a Finnish twin cohort. *Archives of General Psychiatry,* 55, 67-74.

Cantor, S. (1988). *Childhood schizophrenia.* New York: The Guilford Press.

Cardena, E. (1994). The domain of dissociation. In S.J. Lynn and J.W. Rhue (Eds.), *Dissociation: Clinical and theoretical perspectives* (pp. 15-31). New York: The Guilford Press.

Cardena, E., and Spiegel, D. (1989). Dissociative reactions to the Bay Area earthquake. *American Journal of Psychiatry,* 150, 474-478.

Cardino, A.G., Rijsdijk, F.V., Sham, P.C., Murray, R.M., and McGuffin, P. (2002). A twin study of genetic relationships between psychotic symptoms. *American Journal of Psychiatry,* 159, 539-545.

Carlson, E.B., Dalenberg, C., Armstrong, J., Daniels, J.W., Loewenstein, R., and Roth, D. (2001). Multivariate prediction of posttraumatic symptoms in psychiatric inpatients. *Journal of Traumatic Stress,* 14, 549-567.

Carlson, E.B., Putnam, F.W., Ross, C.A., Torem, M., Coons, P., Dill, D.L., Loewenstein, R.J., and Braun, B.G. (1993). Validity of the Dissociative Experiences Scale in screening for multiple personality disorder: A multicenter study. *American Journal of Psychiatry,* 150, 1030-1036.

Carney, R.M., and Jaffe, A.S. (2002). Treatment of depression following acute myocardial infarction. *Journal of the American Medical Association,* 288, 750-751.

Carpenter, W.T. (1984). A perspective on the psychotherapy of schizophrenia project. *Schizophrenia Bulletin,* 10, 599-603.

Carpenter, W.T., Appelbaum, P.S., and Levine, R.J. (2003). The Declaration of Helsinki and clinical trials: A focus on placebo-controlled trials in schizophrenia. *American Journal of Psychiatry,* 160, 356-362.

Cascalenda, N., Perry, J.C., and Looper, K. (2002). Remission in major depressive disorder: A comparison of pharmacotherapy, psychotherapy, and control conditions. *American Journal of Psychiatry,* 159, 1354-1360.

Cheit, R.E. (2002). The legend of Robert Halsey. *Journal of Child Sexual Abuse,* 9, 37-52.

Chovil, I. (2000). First-person account: I and I, dancing fool, challenge you the world to a duel. *Schizophrenia Bulletin,* 26, 745-747.

Chu, J.A. (1998). *Rebuilding shattered lives: The responsible treatment of complex post-traumatic and dissociative disorders.* New York: John Wiley and Sons.

Chu, J.A., and Dill, D.L. (1990). Dissociative symptoms in relation to childhood physical and sexual abuse. *American Journal of Psychiatry,* 147, 887-892.

Chua, S., and Murray, R. (1996). The neurodevelopmental theory of schizophrenia: Evidence concerning structure and neuropsychology. *Annals of Medicine,* 28, 547-551.

Citrome, L., Jaffe, A., Levine, J., and Allingham, B. (2002). Use of mood stabilizers among patients with schizophrenia, 1994-2001. *Psychiatric Services,* 53, 1212.

Cohen, L., Berzoff, J., and Elin, M. (1995). *Dissociative identity disorder: Theoretical and treatment controversies.* Northvale, NJ: Jason Aronson.

Cohen, N.J., and Eichenbaum, H. (1993). *Memory, amnesia, and the hippocampal system.* Cambridge, MA: MIT Press.

Cole, C. (1988). Routine comprehensive inquiry for abuse: A justifiable clinical assessment procedure. *Clinical Social Work Journal,* 16, 33-42.

Cook, E.H. (2000). Genetics of psychiatric disorders: Where have we been and where are we going? *American Journal of Psychiatry,* 157, 1039-1040.

Coons, P.M. (1986). Treatment progress in 20 patients with multiple personality disorder. *Journal of Nervous and Mental Disease,* 174, 715-721.

Coons, P.M. (1994). Confirmation of childhood abuse in child and adolescent cases of multiple personality disorder and dissociative disorder not otherwise specified. *Journal of Nervous and Mental Disease,* 182, 461-464.

Coons, P.M., Bowman, E.S., Kluft, R.P., and Milstein, V. (1991). The cross-cultural occurrence of MPD: Additional cases from a recent survey. *Dissociation,* 4, 124-128.

Coons, P.M., Bowman, E.S., and Milstein, V. (1988). Multiple personality disorder: A clinical investigation of 50 cases. *Journal of Nervous and Mental Disease,* 176, 519-527.

Coons, P.M., and Sterne, A.L. (1986). Initial and follow-up psychological testing on a group of patients with multiple personality disorder. *Psychological Reports,* 58, 43-49.

Courtois, C.A. (1999). *Recollections of sexual abuse: Treatment principles and guidelines.* New York: W.W. Norton.

Craine, L.S., Henson, C.E., Colliver, J.A., and MacLean, D.G. (1988). Prevalence of a history of sexual abuse among female psychiatric patients in a state hospital. *Hospital and Community Psychiatry,* 39, 300-304.

Dallam, S.J. (2002a). Misinformation/disinformation about child sexual abuse. *Journal of Child Sexual Abuse,* 9, 9-36.

Dallam, S.J. (2002b). Science or propaganda? An examination of Rind, Tromovich, and Bauserman. *Journal of Child Sexual Abuse,* 9, 109-134.

Dancu, C.V., Riggs, D.S., Hearst-Ikeda, D., Shoyer, B.G., and Foa, E.B. (1996). Dissociative experiences and posttraumatic stress disorder among female victims of criminal assault and rape. *Journal of Traumatic Stress,* 9, 253-267.

Darves-Bornoz, J.-M., Degiovanni, A., and Gaillard, P. (1995). Why is dissociative identity disorder infrequent in France? *American Journal of Psychiatry,* 152, 1530-1531.

Davidson, J.R.T. (2002). Effect of *Hypericum perforatum* (St. John's wort) in major depressive disorder. *Journal of the American Medical Association,* 287, 1807-1814.

Davis, J.M. (1980). Antipsychotic drugs. In H.I. Kaplan, A.M. Freedman, and B.J. Sadock (Eds.), *Comprehensive textbook of psychiatry,* Volume 3 (pp. 2257-2289). Baltimore: Williams and Wilkins.

de Graff, R., Bijl, R.V., Smit, F., Vollebergh, W.A.M., and Spijker, J. (2002). Risk factors for 12-month comorbidity of mood, anxiety, and substance abuse disorders: Findings from the Netherlands mental health survey and incidence study. *American Journal of Psychiatry,* 159, 620-629.

Dell, P.F. (2002). Dissociative phenomenology of dissociative identity disorder. *Journal of Nervous and Mental Disease,* 190, 10-15.

Dickstein, L.J., Riba, M.B., and Oldham, J.M. (1997). *Repressed memories.* Washington, DC: American Psychiatric Press.

Dill, D., Chu J., Grob, M., and Eisen, S. (1991). The reliability of abuse history reports: A comparison of two inquiry formats. *Comprehensive Psychiatry,* 32, 166-169.

Dixon, L.B., and Lehman, A.F. (1995). Family interventions for schizophrenia. *Schizophrenia Bulletin,* 21, 631-643.

Domash, M.D., and Sparr, L.F. (1982). Post-traumatic stress disorder masquerading as paranoid schizophrenia: A case report. *Military Medicine,* 147, 772-774.

Downs, W., and Miller, B. (1998). Relationships between experiences of parental violence during childhood and women's psychiatric symptomatology. *Journal of Interpersonal Violence,* 13, 438-455.

Dunn, G.E., Paolo, A.M., Ryan, J.J., and Van Fleet, J.N. (1994). Belief in the existence of multiple personality disorder among psychologists and psychiatrists. *Journal of Clinical Psychology,* 50, 454-457.

El-Hage, W., Darves-Bornoz, J.-M., Allilaire, J.-F., and Gaillard, P. (2002). Posttraumatic somatoform dissociation in French psychiatric outpatients. *Journal of Trauma & Dissociation,* 3(3), 59-74.

Ellason, J.W., and Ross, C.A. (1995). Positive and negative symptoms in dissociative identity disorder and schizophrenia. *Journal of Nervous and Mental Disease,* 183(4), 236-241.

Ellason, J.W., and Ross, C.A. (1996). Millon Clinical Multiaxial Inventory-II. Follow-up of patients with dissociative identity disorder. *Psychological Reports,* 78, 707-716.

Ellason, J.W., and Ross, C.A. (1997a). Two-year follow-up of inpatients with dissociative identity disorder. *American Journal of Psychiatry,* 154, 832-839.

Ellason, J.W., and Ross, C.A. (1997b). Childhood trauma and psychiatric symptoms. *Psychological Reports,* 80, 447-450.

Ellason, J.W., Ross, C.A., and Fuchs, D.L. (1995). Assessment of dissociative identity disorder with the Millon Clinical Multiaxial Inventory-II. *Psychological Reports,* 76, 895-905.

Ellason, J.W., Ross, C.A., and Fuchs, D.L. (1996). Lifetime Axis I and II comorbidity and childhood trauma history in dissociative identity disorder. *Psychiatry,* 59, 255-266.

Ellason, J.W., Ross, C.A., Sainton, K. and Mayran, L. (1996). Axis I and II comorbidity and childhood trauma history in chemical dependency. *Bulletin of the Menninger Clinic,* 60, 39-51.

Ellenson, G. (1985). Detecting a history of incest: A predictive syndrome. *Social Casework,* November, 525-532.

Engdahl, B., Dikel, T.N., Eberly, R., and Blank, A. (1998). Comorbidity and course of psychiatric disorders in a community sample of former prisoners of war. *American Journal of Psychiatry,* 155, 1740-1745.

Ensink, B. (1992). *Confusing realities: A study on child sexual abuse and psychiatric symptoms.* Amsterdam, Netherlands: VU University Press.

Erdelyi, M.H. (1996). *The recovery of unconscious memories: Hyperamnesia and reminiscence.* Chicago: University of Chicago Press.

Famularo, R., Kinscherff, R., and Fenton, T. (1992). Psychiatric diagnoses of maltreated children: Preliminary findings. *Journal of the American Academy of Child and Adolescent Psychiatry,* 31, 863-867.

Faraone, S.V., Brown, C.H., Glatt, S.J., and Tsuang, M.T. (2002). Preventing schizophrenia and psychotic behavior: Definitions and methodological issues. *Canadian Journal of Psychiatry,* 47, 527-537.

Feeny, N.C., Zoellner, L.A., and Foa, E.B. (2000). Anger, dissociation, and posttraumatic stress disorder among female assault victims. *Journal of Traumatic Stress,* 13, 89-100.

Feinsilver, D.B., and Gunderson, J.G. (1972). Psychotherapy for schizophrenics—is it indicated? A review of the relevant literature. *Schizophrenia Bulletin,* 1, 11-23.

Feinstein, A. (1989). Posttraumatic stress disorder: A descriptive study supporting DSM-III-R criteria. *American Journal of Psychiatry,* 146, 665-666.

Feldman-Summers, S., and Pope, K.S. (1994). The experience of "forgetting" childhood abuse: A national survey of psychologists. *Journal of Consulting and Clinical Psychology,* 62, 636-639.

Felitti, V.J., Anda, R.F., Nordenberg, D., Williamson, D.F., Spitz, A.M., Edwards, V., Koss, M.P., and Marks, J.S. (1998). Relationship of childhood abuse and household dysfunction to many of the leading causes of death in adults. *American Journal of Preventive Medicine,* 14, 245-258.

Fenton, W.S. (2000). Evolving perspectives on individual psychotherapy for schizophrenia. *Schizophrenia Bulletin,* 26, 47-72.

Fink, D., and Golinkoff, M. (1990). MPD, borderline personality disorder, and schizophrenia: A comparative study of clinical features. *Dissociation,* 3, 127-134.

Fischer, M. (1973). Genetic and environmental factors in schizophrenia. *Acta Psychiatrica Scandinavica,* Supplement 238, 1-153.

Fisher, C. (1945). Amnestic states in war neuroses: The psychogenesis of fugues. *Psychoanalytic Quarterly,* 14, 437-468.

Fisher, C. (1947). The psychogenesis of fugue states. *American Journal of Psychotherapy,* 1, 211-221.

Fisher, C., and Joseph, E.D. (1949). Fugue with loss of personal identity. *Psychoanalytic Quarterly,* 18, 480-493.

Flegal, K.M., Carroll, M.D., Ogden, C.L., and Johnson, C.L. (2002). Prevalence and trends in obesity among U.S. adults, 1999-2000. *Journal of the American Medical Association,* 288, 1723-1727.

Fleming, J., Mullen, P., Sibthorpe, B., and Bammer, G. (1999). The long-term impact of childhood sexual abuse in Australian women. *Child Abuse and Neglect,* 23, 145-159.

Follette, V.M., Ruzek, J.I., and Abueg, F.R. (1998). *Cognitive-behavioral therapies for trauma.* New York: The Guilford Press.

Fontanarosa, P.B. (2002). Obesity research: A call for papers. *Journal of the American Medical Association,* 288, 1772-1773.

Forrest, K.A. (2001). Toward an etiology of dissociative identity disorder: A neurodevelopmental approach. *Consciousness and Cognition,* 10, 259-293.

Frances, A. (1999). The expert consensus panels for schizophrenia. *Journal of Clinical Psychiatry,* (Supplement 11), 1-80.

Freud, S. (1963). Repression (1915). In P. Rief (Ed.), *Freud: General psychological theory* (pp. 104-115). New York: Touchstone Books.

Freyd, J.J. (1996). *Betrayal trauma: The forgetting of child abuse.* Cambridge, MA: Harvard University Press.

Friedl, M.C., and Draijer, N. (2000). Dissociative disorders in Dutch psychiatric inpatients. *American Journal of Psychiatry,* 157, 1012-1013.

Friedman, S., and Harrison, G. (1984). Sexual histories, attitudes, and behavior of schizophrenic and normal women. *Archives of Sexual Behavior,* 13, 555-567.

Fullerton, C.S., Ursano, R.J., Epstein, R.S., Crowley, B., Vance, K.L., Kao, T.-C., and Baum, A. (2000). Peritraumatic dissociation following motor vehicle accidents: Relationship to prior trauma and prior major depression. *Journal of Nervous and Mental Disease,* 188, 267-272.

Gainer, K. (1994). Dissociation and schizophrenia: An historical review of conceptual development and relevant treatment approaches. *Dissociation,* 7, 261-271.

Gast, U., Rodewald, F., Nickel, V., and Emrich, H.M. (2001). Prevalence of dissociative disorders among psychiatric inpatients in a German university clinic. *Journal of Nervous and Mental Disease,* 189, 249-257.

Glassman, A.H., O'Connor, C.M., Califf, R.M., Swedberg, K., Schwartz, P., Bigger, J.T., Krishnan, K.R.R., van Zyl, L.T., Swenson, J.R., Finkel, M.S., et al. (2002). Sertraline treatment of major depression in patients with acute MI or unstable angina. *Journal of the American Medical Association,* 288, 701-709.

Gleaves, D.H. (1996). The sociocognitive model of dissociative identity disorder: A reexamination of the evidence. *Psychological Bulletin,* 120, 42-59.

Gleeson, J., Larsen, T.K., and McGorry, P. (2003). Psychological treatment in pre- and early psychosis. *Journal of the American Academy of Psychoanalysis and Dynamic Psychotherapy,* 31, 229-245.

Goff, D.C. (2002). A 23-year-old man with schizophrenia. *Journal of the American Medical Association,* 287, 3249-3257.

Goff, D., Brotman, A., Kidlon, D., Waites, M., and Amico, E. (1991). Self-reports of childhood abuse in chronically psychotic patients. *Psychiatry Research,* 37, 73-80.

Goldberg, D. (2001). Vulnerability factors for common mental illnesses. *British Journal of Psychiatry,* 178 (Supplement 40), 69-71.

Goldfarb, B. (1992). Under pressure. *AMA News,* November, pp. 23-24.

Goodman, L.A., Thompson, K.M., Weinfurt, K., Corl, S., Acker, P., Mueser, K.T., and Rosenberg, S.D. (1997). Reliability of reports of violent victimization and posttraumatic stress disorder among men and women with serious mental illness. *Journal of Traumatic Stress,* 12, 587-599.

Gottdiener, W.H., and Haslam, N. (2003). A critique of the methods and conclusions in the PORT report. *Journal of the American Academy of Psychoanalysis and Dynamic Psychotherapy,* 31, 191-208.

Gottesman, I.I. (1991). *Schizophrenia genesis: The origins of madness.* New York: W.H. Freeman.

Greenberg, J. (1964). *I never promised you a rose garden.* New York: Signet.

Greenblat, L. (2000). First-person account: Understanding health as a continuum. *Schizophrenia Bulletin,* 26, 243-245.

Hamner, M.B., Frueh, C., Ulmer, H.G., Huber, M.G., Twomey, T.J., Tyson, C., and Arana, G.W. (2000). Psychotic features in chronic posttraumatic stress disorder and schizophrenia. *Journal of Nervous and Mental Disease,* 188, 217-221.

Haugen, M.C., and Castillo, R.J. (1999). Unrecognized dissociation in psychotic outpatients and implications of ethnicity. *Journal of Nervous and Mental Disease,* 187, 751-754.

Heads, T., Taylor, P., and Leese, M. (1997). Childhood experiences of patients with schizophrenia and a history of violence: A special hospital sample. *Criminal and Behavioral Mental Health,* 7, 117-130.

Heim, C., and Nemeroff, C.B. (1999). The impact of early adverse experiences on brain systems involved in the pathophysiology of anxiety and affective disorders. *Biological Psychiatry,* 46, 1509-1522.

Heins, T., Gray, A., and Tennant, M. (1990). Persisting hallucinations following childhood sexual abuse. *Australia and New Zealand Journal of Psychiatry,* 24, 561-565.

Herman, J.L., and Schatzow, E. (1987). Recovery and verification of memories of childhood sexual trauma. *Psychoanalytic Psychology,* 4, 1-14.

Herz, M.I., Liberman, R.P., Lieberman, J.A., Marder, S.R., McGlashan, T.H., Wyatt, R.J., and Wang, P. (1997). Practice guidelines for the treatment of patients with schizophrenia. *American Journal of Psychiatry,* 154(4), 1-63.

Hilgard, E.R. (1977). *Divided consciousness: Multiple controls in human thought and action.* New York: John Wiley and Sons.

Hilgard, E.R. (1994). Neodissociation theory. In S.J. Lynn and J.W. Rhue (Eds.), *Dissociation: Clinical and theoretical perspectives* (pp. 32-51). New York: The Guilford Press.

Hillman, R.G. (1981). The psychopathology of being held hostage. *American Journal of Psychiatry,* 138, 1193-1197.

Hirsch, S.J., and Hollender, M.H. (1969). Hysterical psychosis: Clarification of a concept. *American Journal of Psychiatry,* 125, 909-915.

Hoch, A. (1911). On some of the mental mechanisms in demetia praecox. In A. Meyer, S.E. Jellitt, and A. Hoch (Eds.), *Dementia praecox,* (pp. 51-71). Boston: Gorham Press.

Hollender, M.H., and Hirsch, S.J. (1964). Hysterical psychosis. *American Journal of Psychiatry,* 120, 1066-1074.

Holzinger, A., Loffler, W., Muller, P., Priebe, S., and Angermeyer, M.C. (2002). Subjective illness theory and antipsychotic medication compliance by patients with schizophrenia. *Journal of Nervous and Mental Disease,* 190, 597-603.

Honig, A., Romme, M., Ensink, B., Escher, S., Pennings, M., and De Vies, M. (1998). Auditory hallucinations: A comparison between patients and nonpatients. *Journal of Nervous and Mental Disease,* 186, 646-651.

Horen, S.A., Leichner, P.P., and Lawson, J.S. (1995). Prevalence of dissociative symptoms and disorders in an adult psychiatric population in Canada. *Canadian Journal of Psychiatry,* 40, 185-191.

Huber, M. (1995). *Multiple personlichkeiten.* Frankfurt: Fischer Taschenbuch Verlag.

International Society for the Study of Dissociation (1997). *Guidelines for treating dissociative identity disorder (multiple personality disorder) in adults.* Skokie, IL: International Society for the Study of Dissociation.

Irwin, H., Green, M., and Marsh, P. (1999). Dysfunction in smooth pursuit eye movements and history of childhood trauma. *Perceptual and Motor Skills,* 89, 1230-1236.

Ito, Y., Teicher, M., Gold, C., Harper, D., Magnus, E., and Gelbard, H. (1993). Increased prevalence of electrophysiological abnormalities in children with psychological, physical, and sexual abuse. *Journal of Neuropsychiatry,* 5, 401-408.

Jacobson, A. (1989). Physical and sexual assault histories among psychiatric outpatients. *American Journal of Psychiatry,* 146, 755-758.

Jacobson, A., and Herald, C. (1990). The relevance of childhood sexual abuse to adult psychiatric inpatient care. *Hospital and Community Psychiatry,* 41, 154-158.

Jacobson, A., and Richardson, B. (1987). Assault experiences of 100 psychiatric inpatients: Evidence of the need for routine inquiry. *American Journal of Psychiatry,* 144, 508-513.

Janet, P. (1965 [1907]). *The major symptoms of hysteria.* New York: Hafner.

Janet, P. (1977 [1901]). *The mental state of hystericals.* Washington, DC: University Publications of America.

Jauch, D.A., and Carpenter, W.T. (1988a). Reactive psychosis I: Does the pre-DSM-III-R concept define a third psychosis? *Journal of Nervous and Mental Disease,* 176, 72-81.

Jauch, D.A., and Carpenter, W.T. (1988b). Reactive psychosis II: Does DSM-II-R define a third psychosis? *Journal of Nervous and Mental Disease,* 176, 82-86.

Jay, J. (2001). Don Jackson's "A critique of the literature on the genetics of schizophrenia": A reappraisal after 40 years. *General Sociology and General Psychology Monographs,* 127, 27-57.

Jeffries, J.J. (1977). The trauma of being psychotic: A neglected element in the management of chronic schizophrenia. *Canadian Psychiatric Association Journal,* 22, 199-206.

Jibson, M.D., and Tandon, R. (1998). New atypical antipsychotic medications. *Journal of Psychiatric Research,* 32, 215-228.

Jones, P., Rodgers, B., Murray, R., and Marmont, M. (1994). Child developmental risk factors for adult schizophrenia in the British 1946 birth cohort. *Lancet,* 344, 1398-1402.

Joober, R., Boksa, P., Benkelfat, C., and Rouleau, G. (2002). Genetics of schizophrenia: From animal models to clinical studies. *Journal of Psychiatry and Neuroscience,* 27, 336-347.

Jordan, J.C. (1995). First-person account: Schizophrenia—adrift in an anchorless reality. *Schizophrenia Bulletin,* 21, 501-503.

Kantor, R.E., and Herron, W.G. (1966). *Reactive and process schizophrenia.* Palo Alto: CA: Science and Behavior Books.

Karon, B. (1999). The tragedy of schizophrenia. *General Psychologist,* 34, 1-12.

Kasper, S., and Muller-Spahn, F. (2000). Review of quetiapine and its clinical applications in schizophrenia. *Expert Opinion on Pharmacotherapy,* 1, 783-801.

Kaufman, M.L., Kimble, M.O., Kaloupek, D.G., McTeague, L.M., Bachrach, P., Forti, A.M., and Keane, T.M. (2002). Peritraumatic dissociation and physiological response to trauma-relevant stimuli in Vietnam combat veterans with post-traumatic stress disorder. *Journal of Nervous and Mental Disease,* 190, 167-174.

Kay, S.R., Opler, L.A., and Fiszbein, A. (1994). *Positive and negative syndrome scale manual.* North Tonawanda, NY: Multi-Health Systems.

Kendler, K.S. (1998). The genetics of schizophrenia: Toward the identification of individual susceptibility loci. Dean Award Lecture, American College of Psychiatrists Annual Meeting, San Juan, Puerto Rico, February 21.

Kendler, K.S., Bulik, C.M., Silberg, J., Hettma, J.M., Myers, J., and Prescott, C.A. (2000). Childhood sexual abuse and adult psychiatric and substance use disorders in women. *Archives of General Psychiatry,* 57, 953-959.

Kendler, K.S., Spitzer, R.L., and Williams, J.B.W. (1990). Differential diagnosis of schizophrenia and multiple personality disorder, reply to Rathbun and Rustagi. *American Journal of Psychiatry, 147*, 375.

Kennedy, S., McIntyre, R., Fallu, A., and Lam, R. (2002). Pharmacotherapy to sustain the fully remitted state. *Journal of Psychiatry and Neuroscience, 27*, 269-280.

Kety, S., Rosenthal, D., Wender, P., and Schulsinger, F. (1968). The types and prevalence of mental illness in the biological and adoptive families of schizophrenics. In D. Rosenthal and S. Kety (Eds.), *The transmission of schizophrenia* (pp. 345-362). Oxford: Oxford University Press.

Khan, A., Warner, H.A., and Brown, W.A. (2000). Symptom reduction and suicide risk in patients treated with placebo in antidepressant clinical trials: An analysis of the Food and Drug Administration database. *Archives of General Psychiatry, 57*, 311-317.

Kihlstrom, J.F. (1994). One hundred years of hysteria. In S.J. Lynn and J.W. Rhue (Eds.), *Dissociation: Clinical and theoretical perspectives* (pp. 365-394). New York: The Guilford Press.

Kind, H. (1966). The psychogenesis of schizophrenia. *British Journal of Psychiatry, 112*, 333-349.

Kinderman, P., Cooke, A., and Bentall, R. (2000). *Recent advances in understanding mental illness and psychotic experiences*. Leicester, UK: British Psychological Society.

Kingdon, D.G., and Turkington, D. (1994). *Cognitive-behavioral therapy of schizophrenia*. New York: The Guilford Press.

Kinon, B.J., Roychowdhury, S.M., Milton, D.R., and Hill, A.L. (2002). Effective resolution with olanzapine of acute presentation of behavioral agitation and positive psychotic symptoms in schizophrenia. *Journal of Clinical Psychiatry, 62* (Supplement 2), 17-21.

Klein, M.L., and Doane, B.K. (1994). *Psychological concepts and dissociative disorders*. Hillsdale, NJ: Erlbaum.

Kluft, R.P. (1984). Treatment of multiple personality disorder. *Psychiatric Clinics of North America, 7*, 9-29.

Kluft, R.P. (1985). *Childhood antecedents of multiple personality disorder*. Washington, DC: American Psychiatric Press.

Kluft, R.P. (1987). First-rank symptoms as a diagnostic clue to multiple personality disorder. *American Journal of Psychiatry, 144*, 293-298.

Kluft, R.P. (1998). Reflections on the traumatic memories of dissociative identity disorder patients. In S.J. Lynn and K.M. McConkey (Eds.), *Truth in memory* (pp. 304-322). New York: The Guilford Press.

Kluft, R.P., and Fine, C.G. (1993). *Clinical perspectives on multiple personality disorder*. Washington, DC: American Psychiatric Press.

Knudsen, H., Draijer, N., Haselrud, J., Boe, T., and Boon, S. (1995). Dissociative disorders in Norwegian psychiatric inpatients. Paper presented at the spring meeting of the International Society for the Study of Dissociation, Amsterdam, Netherlands, May.

Koopman, C., Classen, C., and Spiegel, D. (1994). Predictors of posttraumatic stress symptoms among survivors of the Oakland/Berkeley, Calif., firestorm. *American Journal of Psychiatry,* 151, 888-894.

Koopman, C., Classen, C., and Spiegel, D. (1996). Dissociative responses in the immediate aftermath of the Oakland/Berkeley firestorm. *Journal of Traumatic Stress,* 9, 521-540.

Kringlen, E. (1967). *Heredity and environment in the functional psychoses,* Volumes I and II. Oslo, Norway: Universitesforlaget.

Krippner, S., and Powers, S.M. (1997). *Broken images, broken selves: Dissociative narratives in clinical practice.* Washington, DC: Brunner/Mazel.

Krystal, J.H., Bremner, J.D., Southwick, S.M., and Charney, D.S. (1998). The emerging neurobiology of dissociation: Implications for treatment of posttraumatic stress disorder. In J.D. Bremner and C.R. Marmar (Eds.), *Trauma, memory, and dissociation* (pp. 321-363). Washington, DC: American Psychiatric Press.

Kuhn, T. (1962). *The structure of scientific revolutions.* Chicago: University of Chicago Press.

Kunugi, H., Nanko, S., and Murray, R. (2001). Obstetric complications and schizophrenia: Prenatal underdevelopment and subsequent neurodevelopmental impairment. *British Journal of Psychiatry,* 178, 25-29.

Laddis, A., Dell, P.F., Ellason, J.W., Cotton, M., Fridley, D., and Lamb, T. (2001). A comparison of the dissociative experiences of patients with schizophrenia and patients with DID. Paper presented at the Eighteenth International Fall Conference of the International Society for the Study of Dissociation, New Orleans, December 4.

Lalonde, J.K., Hudson, J.L., Gigante, R.A., and Pope, H.G. (2001). Canadian and American psychiatrists' attitudes toward dissociative disorder diagnoses. *Canadian Journal of Psychiatry,* 46, 407-412.

Lalonde, J.K., Hudson, J.I., and Pope, H.G. (2002). Reply to Ross, re: Canadian and American psychiatrists' attitudes toward dissociative disorder diagnoses. *Canadian Journal of Psychiatry,* 47, 282-283.

Lanius, R.A., Williamson, P.C., and Menon, R.S. (2002). Neuroimaging of hyperarousal and dissociative states in posttraumatic stress disorder. *Bulletin of the Canadian Psychiatric Association,* 34, 22-25.

Larsen, T.K., Bechdolf, A., and Birchwood, M. (2003). Cognitive-behavioral treatment in pre-psychosis and in nonresponders. *Journal of the American Academy of Psychoanalysis and Dynamic Psychotherapy,* 31, 209-228.

Latz, T.T., Kramer, S.I., and Hughes, D.L. (1995). Multiple personality disorder among female inpatients in a state hospital. *American Journal of Psychiatry,* 152, 1343-1348.

Leavitt, F. (1997). False attribution of suggestibility to explain recovered memory of childhood sexual abuse following extended amnesia. *Child Abuse and Neglect,* 21, 265-272.

Lecrubier, Y., Clerc, G., Didi, R., and Kieser, M. (2002). Efficacy of St. John's wort extract WS 5570 in major depression: A double-blind, placebo-controlled trial. *American Journal of Psychiatry,* 159, 1361-1366.

Leeper, O.M., Page, B., and Hendricks, D.E. (1992). The prevalence of dissociative disorders in a drug and alcohol abusing population of a residential treatment facility in a military medical center. (Unpublished manuscript).

Lehman, A.F. (1995). Vocational rehabilitation in schizophrenia. *Schizophrenia Bulletin,* 21, 645-656.

Lehman, A.F., Carpenter, W.T., Goldman, H.H., and Steinwachs, D.M. (1995). Treatment outcomes in schizophrenia: Implications for practice, policy, and research. *Schizophrenia Bulletin,* 21, 669-675.

Lehman, A.F., and Steinwachs, D.M. (1998). Translating research into practice: The Schizophrenia Patient Outcomes Research Team (PORT) treatment recommendations. *Schizophrenia Bulletin,* 24, 1-10.

Lehman, A.F., and Steinwachs, D.M. (2003). Lessons learned from the Patient Outcomes Research Team (PORT) report. *Journal of the American Academy of Psychoanalysis and Dynamic Psychotherapy,* 31, 141-154.

Lehman, A.F., Thompson, J.W., Dixon, L.B., and Scott, J.E. (1995). Schizophrenia treatment outcomes research—editors' introduction. *Schizophrenia Bulletin,* 21, 561-566.

Levitan, R.D., Parikh, S.V., Lesage, A.D., Hegadoren, K.M., Adams, M., Kennedy, S.H., and Goering, P.N. (1998). Major depression in individuals with a history of childhood physical or sexual abuse: Relationship to neurovegetative features, mania, and gender. *American Journal of Psychiatry,* 155, 1746-1752.

Lilienfeld, S.O., Lynn, S.J., Kirsch, I., Chaves, J.F., Sarbin, T.R., Ganaway, G.K., and Powell, R.A. (1999). Dissociative identity disorder and the sociocognitive model: Recalling the lessons of the past. *Psychological Bulletin,* 125, 507-523.

Linehan, M. (1993). *Cognitive behavioral treatment for borderline personality disorder.* New York: The Guilford Press.

Linehan, M.M., Armstrong, H.E., Suarez, A., Allmon, D., and Heard, H.L. (1991). Cognitive-behavioral treatment of chronically parasuicidal borderline patients. *Archives of General Psychiatry,* 48, 1060-1064.

Liotti, G. (1992). Disorganized/disoriented attachment in the etiology of dissociative disorders. *Dissociation,* 5, 196-204.

Lipschitz, D., Winegar, R., Nicolaou, A., Hartnick, E., Wolfson, M., and Southwick, S. (1999). Perceived abuse and neglect as risk factors for suicidal behavior in adolescent inpatients. *Journal of Nervous and Mental Disease,* 187, 32-39.

Livingston, R. (1987). Sexually and physically abused children. *Journal of the American Academy of Child and Adolescent Psychiatry,* 26, 413-415.

Loewenstein, R.J. (1993). Psychogenic amnesia and psychogenic fugue: A comprehensive review. In D. Spiegel (Ed.), *Dissociative disorders: A clinical review* (pp. 45-78). Lutherville, MD: Sidran Press.

Loewenstein, R.J. (1996). Dissociative amnesia and dissociative fugue. In L.K. Michelson and W.J. Ray (Eds.), *Handbook of dissociation: Theoretical, empirical and clinical perspectives* (pp. 307-363). New York: Plenum.

Loewenstein, R.J. (2002). Another view: Diagnosis and treatment of iatrogenic and factitious disorder. *The International Society for the Study of Dissociation News,* 20, 6-9, 14.

Loftus, E.F. (1993). The reality of repressed memories. *American Psychologist,* 48, 518-537.

Loftus, E.F., Polonsky, S., and Fullilove, M.T. (1994). Memories of childhood sexual abuse: Remembering and repressing. *Psychology of Women Quarterly,* 18, 67-84.

Lundberg-Love, P., Marmon, S., Ford, K., Geffner, R., and Peacock, L. (1992). The long-term consequences of childhood incestuous victimization upon adult women's psychological symptomatology. *Journal of Child Sexual Abuse,* 1, 81-102.

Lundy, M.S. (1992). Psychosis-induced posttraumatic stress disorder. *American Journal of Psychotherapy,* 46, 485-491.

Lynn, S.J., and McConkey, K.M. (1998). *Truth in memory.* New York: The Guilford Press.

Lynn, S.J., and Rhue, J.W. (1994). *Dissociation: Clinical and theoretical perspectives.* New York: The Guilford Press.

Lysaker, P.H., Meyer, P.S., Evans, J.D., Clements, C.A., and Marks, K.A. (2001). Childhood sexual trauma and psychosocial functioning in adults with schizophrenia. *Psychiatric Services,* 52, 1485-1488.

Macmillan, H.L., Fleming, J.E., Steiner, D.L., Lin, E., Boyle, M.H., Jamieson, E., Duku, E.K., Walsh, C.A., Wong, M.Y.-Y., and Beardslee, W.R. (2001). Childhood abuse and lifetime psychopathology in a community sample. *American Journal of Psychiatry,* 158, 1878-1883.

Maercker, A., Beaducel, A., and Schutzwohl, M. (2000). Trauma severity and initial reactions as precipitating factors for posttraumatic stress symptoms and chronic dissociation in former political prisoners. *Journal of Traumatic Stress,* 13, 651-660.

Mai, F. (1995). Psychiatrists' attitudes to multiple personality disorder: A questionnaire survey. *Canadian Journal of Psychiatry,* 40, 154-157.

Malaspina, D., Goetz, R., Harkavy, F., Kaufman, C., Faraone, S., Tsuang, M., Cloninger, C., Nurnberger, J., and Blehar, M. (2001). Traumatic brain injury and schizophrenia in members of schizophrenia and bipolar disorder pedigrees. *American Journal of Psychiatry,* 158, 440-446.

Malla, A.K., and Norman, R.M.G. (1992). Relationship of major life events and daily stressors to symptomatology in schizophrenia. *Journal of Nervous and Mental Disease,* 180, 664-667.

Mallett, B.L., and Gold, S. (1964). A pseudo-schizophrenic hysterical syndrome. *British Journal of Medical Psychology,* 37, 59-70.

Malmberg, A., Lewis, G., and Allebeck, P. (1998). Premorbid adjustment and personality in people with schizophrenia. *British Journal of Psychiatry,* 172, 308-313.

March, J.S., Biederman, J., Wolkow, R., Safferman, A., Mardekian, J., Cook, E.H., Cutler, N.R., Dominguez, R., Ferguson, J., Muller, B., et al. (1998). Sertraline in children and adolescents with obsessive-compulsive disorder. *Journal of the American Medical Association,* 280, 1752-1756.

Margison, F. (2003). Evidence-based medicine in psychological treatment. *Journal of the American Academy of Psychoanalysis and Dynamic Psychotherapy,* 31, 177-190.

Markowitsch, H.J., Kessler, J., Van Der Ven, C., Weber-Luxenburger, G., Albers, M., and Heiss, W.-D. (1998). Psychic trauma causing grossly reduced brain metabolism and cognitive function. *Neuropsychologia,* 36, 77-82.

Marmar, C.R., Weiss, D.S., Metzler, T.J., Delucchi, K.L., Best, S.R., and Wentworth, K.A. (1999). Longitudinal course and predictors of continuing distress following critical incident exposure in emergency services personnel. *Journal of Nervous and Mental Disease,* 187, 15-22.

Marmar, C.R., Weiss, D.S., Schlenger, W.E., Fairbank, J.A., Jordan, B.K., Kulka, R.A., and Hough, R.L. (1994). Peritraumatic dissociation and posttraumatic stress in male Vietnam theater veterans. *American Journal of Psychiatry,* 151, 908-913.

Martin, P.A. (1971). Dynamic considerations of the hysterical psychosis. *American Journal of Psychiatry,* 128, 745-748.

Martinez-Taboas, A. (1989). Multiple personality disorder in Puerto Rico: Analysis of fifteen cases. *Dissociation,* 2, 128-131.

Martinez-Taboas, A. (1995). A sociocultural analysis of Merskey's approach. In L. Cohen, J. Berzoff, and M. Elin (Eds.), *Dissociative identity disorder: Theoretical and treatment controversies* (pp. 57-63). Northvale, NJ: Jason Aronson.

Masson, J.M. (1985). *The complete letters of Sigmund Freud to Wilhelm Fleiss 1887-1904.* Cambridge, MA: Belknap Press.

McEvoy, J.P., Scheifler, P.L., and Frances, A. (1999). The expert consensus guidelines series: Treatment of schizophrenia. *Journal of Clinical Psychiatry,* 60 (Supplement 11), 1-80.

McGlashan, T.H., and Nayfack, B. (1988). Psychotherapeutic models and the treatment of schizophrenia: The records of three successive psychotherapists with one patient at Chestnut Lodge for eighteen years. *Psychiatry,* 51, 340-362.

McGorry, P.D., Chanen, A., McCarthy, E., Van Riel, R., McKenzie, D., and Singh, B. (1991). Postraumatic stress disorder following recent-onset psychosis. *Journal of Nervous and Mental Disease,* 179, 253-258.

McGuffin, P., Asherson, P., Owen, M., and Farmer, A. (1994). The strength of the genetic effect: Is there room for an environmental influence in the aetiology of schizophrenia? *British Journal of Psychiatry,* 164, 593-599.

McHugh, P.R. (1997). Foreword. In A. Piper, *Hoax and reality: The bizarre world of multiple personality disorder* (pp. ix-x). Northvale, NJ: Jason Aronson.

McKenna, K., Gordon, C., and Rapaport, J. (1994). Childhood-onset schizophrenia: Timely neurobiological research. *Journal of the American Academy of Child and Adolescent Psychiatry,* 33, 771-781.

Merckelbach, H., Rassin, E., and Muris, P. (2000). Dissociation, schizotypy, and fantasy proneness in undergraduate students. *Journal of Nervous and Mental Disease,* 188, 428-431.

Merskey, H. (1995). The manufacture of personalities: The production of multiple personality disorder. In L. Cohen, J. Berzoff, and M. Elin (Eds.), *Dissociative identity disorder: Theoretical and treatment controversies* (pp. 3-32). Northvale, NJ: Jason Aronson.

Meyer, A. (1911 [1950]). The nature and conception of dementia praecox. In A. Meyer, S.E. Jelliffe, and A. Hoch (Eds.), *Dementia praecox: A monograph.* (pp. 7-18). Boston: Gorham Press.

Meyer, A., Jelliffe, S.E., and Hoch, A. (1911 [1950]). *Dementia praecox: A monograph.* Boston: Gorham Press.

Meyer, H., Taiminen, T., Vuori, T., Aijala, A., and Helenius, H. (1999). Posttraumatic stress disorder symptoms related to psychosis and acute involuntary hospitalization in schizophrenic and delusional patients. *Journal of Nervous and Mental Disease,* 187, 343-352.

Michelson, L.K., and Ray, W.J. (1996). *Handbook of dissociation.* New York: Plenum.

Middleton, W., and Butler, J. (1998). Dissociative identity disorder: An Australian series. *Australia and New Zealand Journal of Psychiatry,* 32, 794-804.

Miller, A.L., Chiles, J.A., Chiles, J.K., Crismon, M.L., Rush, A.J., and Shon, S.P. (1999). The Texas Medication Algorithm Project (TMAP) schizophrenia algorithms. *Journal of Clinical Psychiatry,* 60, 649-657.

Millon, T. (1977). *Millon Clinical Multiaxial Inventory manual.* Minneapolis, MN: National Computer Systems.

Milner, K.K., and Valenstein, M. (2002). A comparison of guidelines for the treatment of schizophrenia. *Psychiatric Services,* 53, 888-892.

Modestin, J., Ebner, G., Juhnghan, M., and Erni, T. (1996). Dissociative experiences and dissociative disorders in acute psychiatric inpatients. *Comprehensive Psychiatry,* 37, 355-361.

Morgan, C.A., Hazlett, G., Wang, S., Richardson, G., Schnurr, P., and Southwick, S.M. (2001). Symptoms of dissociation in humans experiencing acute, uncontrollable stress: A prospective investigation. *American Journal of Psychiatry,* 158, 1239-1247.

Mosher, L.R. (1999). Soteria and other alternatives to acute psychiatric hospitalization. *Journal of Nervous and Mental Disease,* 187, 142-149.

Muenzenmaier, K., Meyer, I., Struening, E., and Ferber, J. (1993). Childhood abuse and neglect among women outpatients with chronic mental illness. *Hospital and Community Psychiatry,* 44, 666-670.

Mueser, K.T., and Berenbaum, H. (1990). Psychodynamic treatment of schizophrenia: Is there a future? *Psychological Medicine,* 20, 253-262.

Mueser, K.T., and Butler, R.W. (1987). Auditory hallucinations in combat-related chronic posttraumatic stress disorder. *American Journal of Psychiatry,* 144, 299-302.

Mueser, K.T., Trumbetta, S.L., Rosenberg, S.D., Vidaver, R., Goodman, L.B., Osher, F.C., Auciello, P.P., and Foy, D.W. (1998). Trauma and posttraumatic stress disorder in severe mental illness. *Journal of Consulting and Clinical Psychology,* 66, 493-499.

Mullen, P., Martin, J., Anderson, J., Romans, S., and Herbison, P. (1993). Child sexual abuse and mental health in adult life. *British Journal of Psychiatry,* 163, 721-732.

Murphy, P. (1994). Dissociative experiences and dissociative disorders in a nonclinical university group. *Dissociation,* 7, 28-34.

Nelson, M.D., Saykin, A.J., Flashman, L.A., and Riordan, H.J. (1998). Hippocampal volume reduction in schizophrenia as assessed by magnetic resonance imaging. *Archives of General Psychiatry,* 55, 433-440.

Neumann, S., Grimes, K., Walker, E., and Baum, K. (1995). Developmental pathways to schizophrenia: Behavioral subtypes. *Journal of Abnormal Psychology,* 104, 558-566.

Newport, D.J., Stowe, Z.N., and Nemeroff, C.B. (2002). Parental depression: Animal models of an adverse life event. *American Journal of Psychiatry,* 159, 1265-1283.

Nijenhuis, E.R.S. (1999). *Somatoform dissociation: Phenomena, measurement, and theoretical issues.* Assen, Netherlands: Van Gorcum.

Nijenhuis, E.R.S., Ehling, T., and Krikke, A. (2002). Hippocampal volume in florid and recovered DID, DDNOS, and healthy controls: Three MRI studies. Paper presented at the International Society for the Study of Dissociation Nineteenth International Fall Conference, Baltimore, Maryland, November 11.

Nijenhuis, E.R.S., van der Hart, O., and Steele, K. (2002). The emerging psychobiology of trauma-related dissociation and dissociative disorders. *Biological Psychiatry,* 21, 1081-1098.

Norman, R., and Malla, A. (1993a). Stressful life events and schizophrenia: I. A review of the research. *British Journal of Psychiatry,* 162, 161-166.

Norman, R., and Malla, A. (1993b). Stressful life events and schizophrenia: II. Conceptual and methodological issues. *British Journal of Psychiatry,* 162, 166-174.

Norton, J. (1982). Expressed emotion, affective style, voice tone and communication deviance as predictors of offspring schizophrenia spectrum disorders. Unpublished doctoral dissertation, University of California, Los Angeles.

Noyes, R., Hoenk, P.R., Kuperman, S., and Slymen, D.J. (1977). Depersonalization in accident victims and psychiatric patients. *Journal of Nervous and Mental Disease,* 164, 401-407.

Ofshe, R., and Watters, E. (1994). *Making monsters: False memories, psychotherapy, and sexual hysteria.* New York: Charles Scribner's Sons.

Ogden, C.L., Flegal, K.M., Carroll, M.D., and Johnson, C.L. (2002). Prevalence and trends in overweight among U.S. children and adolescents, 1999-2000. *Journal of the American Medical Association,* 288, 1728-1732.

Oquendo, M.A., Kamali, M., Ellis, S.P., Gruenbaum, M.F., Malone, K.M., Brodsky, B.S., Sackheim, H.A., and Mann, J.L. (2002). Adequacy of antidepressant treatment after discharge and the occurrence of suicidal acts in major depression: A prospective study. *American Journal of Psychiatry,* 159, 1746-1751.

Overall, J.E., and Gorham, D.R. (1988). The Brief Psychiatric Rating Scale (BPRS): Recent developments in ascertainment and scaling. *Psychopharmacology Bulletin,* 24, 97-99.

Pain, C. (2002). PTSD and comorbidity or disorder of extreme stress not otherwise specified. *Bulletin of the Canadian Psychiatric Association,* 34, 12-14.

Palmer, R., Bramble, D., Metcalfe, M., Oppenheimer, R., and Smith, J. (1994). Childhood sexual experiences with adults: Adult male psychiatric patients and general practice attenders. *British Journal of Psychiatry,* 165, 675-679.

Pam, A. (1995). Biological psychiatry: Science or pseudoscience? In C.A. Ross and A. Pam (Eds.), *Pseudoscience in biological psychiatry* (pp. 7-84). New York: John Wiley and Sons.

Pam, A., Kemker, S.S., Ross, C.A., and Golden, R. (1996). The "equal environments assumption" in MZ-DZ twin comparisons: An untenable premise of psychiatric genetics. *Acta Genetica Medica Gemellology,* 45, 349-360.

Pettigrew, J., and Burcham, B. (1997). Effects of childhood sexual abuse in adult female psychiatric patients. *Australia and New Zealand Journal of Psychiatry,* 31, 208-213.

Pezdek, K., and Banks, W.P.P. (1996). *The recovered memory/false memory debate.* New York: Academic Press.

Pinals, D.A., and Breier, A. (1997). Schizophrenia. In A. Tasman, J. Kay, and J.A. Lieberman (Eds.), *Psychiatry* (pp. 927-965). Philadelphia: W.B. Saunders.

Pincus, H.A., Rush, A.J., First, M.B., and McQueen, L.E. (2000). *Handbook of psychiatric measures.* Washington, DC: American Psychiatric Association.

Pinto, P.A., and Gregory, R.J. (1995). Posttraumatic stress disorder with psychotic features. *American Journal of Psychiatry,* 52, 471-472.

Piper, A. (1997). *Hoax and reality: The bizarre world of multiple personality disorder.* Northvale, NJ: Jason Aronson.

Ploghaus, A., Tracey, I., Gati, J.S., Clare, S., Menon, R.S., Matthews, P.M., and Rawlins, J.N.P. (1999). Dissociating pain from its anticipation in the human brain. *Science,* 284, 1979-1981.

Pope, C.A., and Kwapil, T.R. (2000). Dissociative experiences in hypothetically psychosis-prone college students. *Journal of Nervous and Mental Disease,* 188, 530-536.

Pope, H.G., and Hudson, J.I. (1992). Is childhood sexual abuse a risk factor for bulimia nervosa? *American Journal of Psychiatry,* 149, 241-248.

Pope, H.G., Oliva, P.S., Hudson, J.I., Bodkin, J.A., and Gruber, A.J. (1999). Attitudes towards DSM-IV dissociative disorders diagnoses among board-certified American psychiatrists. *American Journal of Psychiatry,* 156, 321-323.

Pope, K.S. (1996). Memory, abuse, and science: Questioning claims about the false memory syndrome epidemic. *American Psychologist,* 51, 957-974.

Pope, K.S. (1997). Science as careful questioning: Are claims of a false memory epidemic based on empirical evidence? *American Psychologist,* 52, 997-1006.

Putnam, F.W. (1989). *Diagnosis and treatment of multiple personality disorder.* New York: The Guilford Press.

Putnam, F.W. (1995). Resolved: Multiple personality disorder is an individually and socially created artifact. Negative. *Journal of the American Academy of Child and Adolescent Psychiatry,* 34, 960-962; Rebuttal, 963.

Putnam, F.W. (1997). *Dissociation in children and adolescents.* New York: The Guilford Press.

Putnam, F.W., Guroff, J.J., Silberman, E.K., Barban, L., and Post, R.M. (1986). The clinical phenomenology of multiple personality disorder: Review of 100 cases. *Journal of Clinical Psychiatry,* 47, 285-293.

Putnam, F.W., and Loewenstein, R.J. (1993). Treatment of multiple personality disorder: A survey of current practices. *American Journal of Psychiatry,* 150, 1048-1052.

Quen, J.M. (1986). *Split minds split brains: Historical and current perspectives.* New York: New York University Press.

Rathbun, J.M., and Rustagi, P.K. (1990). Differential diagnosis of schizophrenia and multiple personality disorder. *American Journal of Psychiatry,* 147, 375.

Read, J. (1997). Child abuse and psychosis: A literature review and implications for professional practice. *Professional Psychology: Research and Practice,* 28, 448-456.

Read, J. (1998). Child abuse and severity of disturbance among adult psychiatric inpatients. *Child Abuse and Neglect,* 22, 359-368.

Read, J. (2001). The relationship between child abuse and schizophrenia: Causal, contributory or coincidental? Paper presented at Royal Australian and New Zealand College of Psychiatrists Thirty-Sixth Annual Congress, Canberra.

Read, J., Agar, K., Argyle, N., and Aderhold, V. (in press). Sexual and physical abuse during childhood and adulthood as predictors of hallucinations, delusions and thought disorder. *Psychology and Psychotherapy: Theory, Research and Practice.*

Read, J., Agar, K., Barker-Collo, S., Davies, E., and Moskowitz, A. (2001). Assessing suicidality in adults: Integrating childhood trauma as a major risk factor. *Professional Psychology: Research and Practice,* 32, 367-372.

Read, J., and Argyle, N. (1999). Hallucinations, delusions, and thought disorder among adult psychiatric inpatients with a history of child abuse. *Psychiatric Services,* 50, 1467-1472.

Read, J., and Argyle, N. (2000). A question of abuse. *Psychiatric Services,* 51, 534-535.

Read, J., Mosher, L., and Bentall, R. (Eds.) (2004). *Models of madness: Psychological, social and biological approaches to schizophrenia* (pp. 101-113). London: Brunner-Routledge.

Read, J., Perry, B.D., Moskowitz, A., and Connolly, J. (2001). The contribution of early traumatic events to schizophrenia in some patients: A traumagenic neurodevelopmental model. *Psychiatry: Interpersonal and Biological Processes,* 64, 319-345.

Read, J., and Ross, C.A. (2003). Psychological trauma and psychosis. *Journal of the American Academy of Psychoanalysis and Dynamic Psychiatry,* 31, 247-268.

Rector, N.A., and Beck, A.T. (2001). Cognitive behavioral therapy for schizophrenia: An empirical review. *Journal of Nervous and Mental Disease,* 189, 278-287.

Rector, N.A., and Beck, A.T. (2002). Cognitive therapy for schizophrenia: From conceptualization to intervention. *Canadian Journal of Psychiatry,* 47, 39-48.

Richman, J., and White, H. (1970). A family view of hysterical psychosis. *American Journal of Psychiatry,* 127, 280-285.

Rifkin, A., Ghisalbert, D., Dimatou, S., Jin, C., and Sethi, M. (1998). Dissociative identity disorder in psychiatric inpatients. *American Journal of Psychiatry,* 155, 844-845.

Rivera, M. (1996). *More alike than different: Treating severely dissociative trauma survivors*. Toronto: University of Toronto Press.

Robins, L. (1966). *Deviant children grown up*. New York: Williams and Wilkins.

Rodnick, E., Goldstein, M., Lewis, J., and Doane, J. (1984). Parental communication style, affect, and role as precursors of offspring schizophrenia-spectrum disorders. In N. Watt, E. Anthony, L. Wynne, and J. Rolf (Eds.), *Children at risk for schizophrenia* (pp. 81-92). Cambridge: Cambridge University Press.

Rose, S. (1991). Acknowledging abuse backgrounds of intensive case management clients. *Community Mental Health Journal, 27*, 255-263.

Rose, S., Peabody, C., and Stratigeas, B. (1991). Undetected abuse among intensive case management clients. *Hospital and Community Psychiatry, 42*, 499-503.

Rosenbaum, M. (1980). The role of the term schizophrenia in the decline of diagnoses of multiple personality. *Archives of General Psychiatry, 37*, 1383-1385.

Rosenberg, S.I., Mueser, K.T., Friedman, M.J., Gorman, P.G., Drake, R.E., Vidaver, R.M., Torrey, W.C., and Jankowski, M.K. (2001). Developing effective treatments for posttraumatic disorders among people with severe mental illness. *Psychiatric Services, 52*, 1453-1661.

Rosenberg, S., Mueser, K., Jankowski, M.K., and Hamblen, J. (2002). Trauma exposure and PTSD in people with severe mental illness. *PTSD Research Quaterly, 13*, 1-4.

Rosenfarb, I., Nuechterlein, K., Goldstein, M., and Subotnik, K. (2000). Neurocognitive vulnerability, interpersonal criticism, and the emergence of unusual thinking by schizophrenic patients during family transactions. *Archives of General Psychiatry, 57*, 1174-1179.

Ross, C.A. (1984). Diagnosis of multiple personality during hypnosis: A case report. *International Journal of Clinical and Experimental Hypnosis, 32*, 222-235.

Ross, C.A. (1985). DSM-III: Problems in diagnosing partial forms of multiple personality disorder. *Journal of the Royal Society of Medicine, 75*, 933-936.

Ross, C.A. (1986). Biological tests for mental illness: Their use and misuse. *Biological Psychiatry, 21*, 431-435.

Ross, C.A. (1989). *Multiple personality disorder: Diagnosis, clinical features, and treatment*. New York: John Wiley and Sons.

Ross, C.A. (1991). Epidemiology of multiple personality and dissociation. *Psychiatric Clinics of North America, 14*, 503-517.

Ross, C.A. (1994). *The Osiris complex: Case studies in multiple personality disorder*. Toronto: University of Toronto Press.

Ross, C.A. (1995). *Satanic ritual abuse: Principles of treatment*. Toronto: University of Toronto Press.

Ross, C.A. (1997). *Dissociative identity disorder: Diagnosis, clinical features, and treatment of multiple personality* (Second edition). New York: John Wiley and Sons.

Ross, C.A. (1999). The dissociative disorders. In T. Millon, P.P. Blaney, and R. Davis (Eds.), *Oxford textbook of psychopathology* (pp. 466-481). New York: Oxford University Press.

Ross, C.A. (2000a). *BLUEBIRD: Deliberate creation of multiple personality by psychiatrists*. Richardson, TX: Manitou Communications.

Ross, C.A. (2000b). *The trauma model: A solution to the problem of comorbidity in psychiatry*. Richardson, TX: Manitou Communications.

Ross, C.A. (2002). Re: Canadian and American psychiatrists' attitudes toward dissociative disorder diagnoses. *Canadian Journal of Psychiatry*, 47, 282.

Ross, C.A. (in press). Dissociation and psychosis: The need for integration of theory and practice. In J.O. Johannessen and B. Martindale (Eds.), *Schizophrenia and other psychoses: Different stages, different treatment?* New York: Brunner-Routledge.

Ross, C.A., Anderson, G., and Clark, P. (1994). Childhood abuse and positive symptoms of schizophrenia. *Hospital and Community Psychiatry*, 45, 489-491.

Ross, C.A., Anderson, G., Fleisher, W.P., and Norton, G.R. (1991). The frequency of multiple personality disorder among psychiatric inpatients. *American Journal of Psychiatry*, 148, 1717-1720.

Ross, C.A., Anderson, G., Fraser, G.A., Reagor, P., Bjornson, L., and Miller, S.D. (1992). Differentiating multiple personality disorder and dissociative disorder not otherwise specified. *Dissociation*, 5, 87-90.

Ross, C.A., Duffy, C.M.M., and Ellason, J.W. (2002). Prevalence, reliability and validity of dissociative disorders in an inpatient setting. *Journal of Trauma and Dissociation*, 3, 7-17.

Ross, C.A., and Ellason, J.W. (2001). Acute stabilization in an inpatient trauma program. *Journal of Trauma and Dissociation*, 2, 83-87.

Ross, C.A., Heber, S., Norton, G.R., and Anderson, G. (1989). Differences between multiple personality disorder and other diagnostic groups on structured interview. *Journal of Nervous and Mental Disease*, 179, 487-491.

Ross, C.A., Heber, S., Norton, G.R., Anderson, D., Anderson, G., and Barchet, P. (1989). The Dissociative Disorders Interview Schedule: A structured interview. *Dissociation*, 2, 169-189.

Ross, C.A., and Joshi, S. (1992). Schneiderian symptoms and childhood trauma in the general population. *Comprehensive Psychiatry*, 33, 269-273.

Ross, C.A., Joshi, S., and Currie, R.P.P. (1990). Dissociative experiences in the general population. *American Journal of Psychiatry*, 147, 1547-1552.

Ross, C.A., Keyes, B., and Xiao, Z. (2002). Dissociation in China. Paper presented at the Nineteenth International Fall Conference of the International Society for the Study of Dissociation, Baltimore, Maryland, November 9.

Ross, C.A., Miller, S.D., Bjornson, L., Reagor, P., Fraser, G.A., and Anderson, G. (1990). Schneiderian symptoms in multiple personality disorder and schizophrenia. *Comprehensive Psychiatry*, 31, 111-118.

Ross, C.A., Miller, S.D., Reagor, P., Bjornson, L., Fraser, G.A., and Anderson, G. (1990). Structured interview data on 102 cases of multiple personality disorder from four centers. *American Journal of Psychiatry*, 147, 596-601.

Ross, C.A., and Norton, G.R. (1988). Multiple personality disorder patients with a prior diagnosis of schizophrenia. *Dissociation*, 1(2), 39-42.

Ross, C.A., Norton, G.R., and Fraser, G.A. (1989). Evidence against the iatrogenesis of multiple personality disorder. *Dissociation*, 2, 61-65.

Ross, C.A., Norton, G.R., and Wozney, K. (1989). Multiple personality disorder: An analysis of 236 cases. *Canadian Journal of Psychiatry*, 34, 413-418.

Ross, C.A., and Pam, A. (1995). *Pseudoscience in biological psychiatry.* New York: John Wiley and Sons.

Ross, C.A., and Read, J. (2004). Antipsychotic medication—myths and facts. In J. Read and R. Bentall (Eds.), *Models of madness: Psychological, social and biological approaches to schizophrenia* (pp. 101-103). London: Brunner-Routledge.

Ross, C.A., Ryan, L., Voigt, H., and Edie, L. (1991). High and low dissociators in a college student population. *Dissociation, 4,* 147-151.

Ruocchio, P.J. (1989). First-person account: Fighting the fight—the schizophrenic's nightmare. *Schizophrenia Bulletin, 15,* 163-166.

Ruocchio, P.J. (1991). First-person account: The schizophrenic inside. *Schizophrenia Bulletin, 17,* 357-360.

Ryan, L.G. (1988). Prevalence of dissociative disorders and symptoms in a university population. Doctoral thesis, University of Manitoba.

Sanchez-Planell, L., and Diez-Quevedo, C. (2000). *Dissociative states.* Barcelona: Springer-Verlag Iberica.

Sanders, A.R., and Gejman, P.V. (2001). Influential ideas and experimental progress in schizophrenia genetics research. *Journal of the American Medical Association, 285,* 2831-2833.

Sansonnet-Hayden, H., Haley, G., Marriage, K., and Fine, S. (1987). Sexual abuse and psychopathology in hospitalized adolescents. *Journal of the American Academy of Child and Adolescent Psychiatry, 26,* 753-757.

Sapolsky, R.M. (2000). Glucocorticoids and hippocampal atrophy in neuropsychiatric disorders. *Archives of General Pychiatry, 57,* 925-935.

Sapolsky, R.M. (2003). Gene therapy for psychiatric disorders. *American Journal of Psychiatry, 160,* 208-220.

Sar, V., Yargic, I., and Tutkun, H. (1996). Structured interview data on 35 cases of dissociative identity disorder from Turkey. *American Journal of Psychiatry, 153,* 1329-1333.

Sautter, F.J., Brailey, K., Uddo, M.M., Hamilton, M.F., Beard, M.G., and Borges, A.H. (1999). PTSD and comorbid psychotic disorder: Comparison with veterans diagnosed with PTSD or psychotic disorder. *Journal of Traumatic Stress, 12,* 73-88.

Sautter, F.J., Cornwell, J., Johnson, J.J., Wiley, J., and Faraone, S.V. (2002). Family history study of posttraumatic stress disorder with secondary psychotic features. *American Journal of Psychiatry, 159,* 1775-1777.

Saxe, G.N., van der Kolk, B.A., Berkowitz, R., Chinman, G., Hall, K., Lieberg, G., and Schwartz, J. (1993). Dissociative disorders in psychiatric inpatients. *American Journal of Psychiatry, 150,* 1037-1042.

Scheflin, A.W. (2003). Dissociation and the law: Is MPD/DID real to the courts? *International Society for the Study of Dissociation News, 21*(1), 2-4, 12.

Schneider, K. (1959). *General psychopathology.* Hamilton, NY: Grune and Stratton.

Schultz, R.K., Braun, B.G., and Kluft, R.P. (1989). Multiple personality disorder: Phenomenology of selected variables in comparison to major depression. *Dissociation, 2,* 45-51.

Scott, J.E., and Dixon, L.B. (1995a). Assertive community treatment and case management for schizophrenia. *Schizophrenia Bulletin*, 21, 657-668.

Scott, J.E., and Dixon, L.B. (1995b). Psychological interventions for schizophrenia. *Schizophrenia Bulletin*, 21, 621-630.

Scott, R., and Stone, D. (1986). MMPI profile constellations in incest families. *Journal of Consulting and Clinical Psychology*, 54, 364-368.

Sedman, G. (1966a). A comparative study of pseudohallucinations, imagery, and true hallucinations. *British Journal of Psychiatry*, 112, 9-17.

Sedman, G. (1966b). "Inner voices": Phenomenological and clinical aspects. *British Journal of Psychiatry*, 112, 485-490.

Shalev, A.Y., Peri, T., Canetti, L., and Schreiber, S. (1996). Predictors of PTSD in injured trauma survivors: A prospective study. *American Journal of Psychiatry*, 153, 219-225.

Shaner, A., and Eth, S. (1989). Can schizophrenia cause posttraumatic stress disorder? *American Journal of Psychotherapy*, 43, 588-597.

Shaw, K., McFarlane, A., and Bookless, C. (1997). The phenomenology of traumatic reactions to psychotic illness. *Journal of Nervous and Mental Disease*, 185, 434-441.

Shaw, K., McFarlane, A.C., Bookless, C., and Air, T. (2002). The aetiology of postpsychotic posttraumatic stress disorder following a psychotic episode. *Journal of Traumatic Stress*, 15, 39-47.

Silberg, J. (1996). *The dissociative child*. Lutherville, MD: Sidran Press.

Silver, A.L., and Larsen, T.K. (2003). FRONTLINE—The schizophrenic person and the benefit of the psychotherapies—seeking a PORT in the storm. *Journal of the American Academy of Psychoanalysis and Dynamic Psychotherapy*, 31, 1-10.

Silver, R.C., Holman, E.A., McIntosh, D.N., Poulin, M., and Gil-Rivas, V. (2002). Nationwide longitudinal study of psychological response to September 11. *Journal of the American Medical Association*, 288, 1235-1244.

Simpson, M. (1995). Gullible's travels, or the importance of being multiple. In L. Cohen, J. Berzoff, and M. Elin (Eds.), *Dissociative identity disorder: Theoretical and treatment controversies* (pp. 87-134). Northvale, NJ: Jason Aronson.

Singer, J. (1990). *Repression and dissociation: Implications for personality theory, psychopathology, and health*. Chicago: University of Chicago Press.

Siomopoulos, V. (1971). Hysterical psychosis: Psychopathological aspects. *British Journal of Medical Psychology*, 44, 95-100.

Smith, T.E., and Docherty, J.P. (1998). Standards of care and clinical algorithms for treating schizophrenia. *Psychiatric Clinics of North America*, 21, 203-220.

Spanos, N.P. (1996). *Multiple identities and false memories: A sociocognitive perspective*. Washington, DC: American Psychological Association.

Spencer, E., and Campbell, M. (1994). Children with schizophrenia: Diagnosis, phenomenology, and pharmacotherapy. *Schizophrenia Bulletin*, 20, 713-725.

Spiegel, D. (1993). *Dissociative disorders: A clinical review*. Lutherville, MD: Sidran Press.

Spiegel, D. (1994). *Dissociation: Culture, mind, and body*. Washington, DC: American Psychiatric Press.

Spiegel, D. (1997). *Repressed memories*. Washington, DC: American Psychiatric Press.

Spiegel, D., and Butler, L.D. (2002). Acute stress in response to the terrorist attacks on September 11, 2001. *Bulletin of the Canadian Psychiatric Association, 34*, 15-18.

Spiegel, D., and Fink, R. (1979). Hysterical psychosis and hypnotizability. *American Journal of Psychiatry, 136*, 777-781.

Spira, J.L. (1996). *Treating dissociative identity disorder*. San Francisco: Jossey-Bass.

Spitzer, C., Haug, H.-J., and Freyberger, H.J. (1997). Dissociative symptoms in schizophrenic patients with positive and negative symptoms. *Psychopathology, 30*, 67-75.

Spitzer, R.L., Williams, J.B.W., Gibbon, M., and First, M.B. (1990). *Users' guide for the Structured Clinical Interview for DSM-III-R*. Washington, DC: American Psychiatric Press.

Stabenau, J.R., and Pollin, W. (1993). Heredity and environment in schizophrenia, revisited. *Journal of Nervous and Mental Disease, 181*, 290-297.

Startup, M. (1999). Schizotypy, dissociative experiences and childhood abuse: Relationships among self-report measures. *British Journal of Clinical Psychology, 38*, 333-344.

Stein, M.B., Jang, K.L., Taylor, S., Vernon, P.A., and Livesley, W.J. (2002). Genetic and environmental influences on trauma exposure and posttraumatic stress disorder symptoms: A twin study. *American Journal of Psychiatry, 159*, 1675-1681.

Stein, M.B., Kline, N.A., and Matloff, J.L. (2002). Adjunctive olanzepine for SSRI-resistant combat-related PTSD: A double-blind, placebo-controlled study. *American Journal of Psychiatry, 159*, 1777-1779.

Stein, M.B., Koverola, C., Hanna, C., Torchia, M.G., and McClarty, B. (1997). Hippocampal volume in women victimized by childhood trauma. *Psychological Medicine, 27*, 951-959.

Steinberg, M. (1995). *Handbook for the assessment of dissociation: A clinical guide*. Washington, DC: American Psychiatric Press.

Steinberg, M., Cicchetti, D., Buchanan, J., Rakfeldt, J., and Rounsaville, B. (1994). Distinguishing between multiple personality disorder (dissociative identity disorder) and schizophrenia using the structured clinical interview for DSM-IV dissociative disorders. *Journal of Nervous and Mental Disease, 182*, 495-502.

Steinberg, M., Rounsaville, B.J., and Cicchetti, D.V. (1990). The Structured Clinical Interview for DSM-III-R Dissociative Disorders: Preliminary report on a new diagnostic instrument. *American Journal of Psychiatry, 147*, 76-82.

Steingard, S., and Frankel, F.H. (1985). Dissociation and psychotic symptoms. *American Journal of Psychiatry, 142*, 953-955.

Stone, M.H. (1989). The course of borderline personality disorder. In A. Tasman, R.E. Hales, and A.J. Frances (Eds.). *Review of psychiatry*, Volume 8 (pp. 103-122). Washington, DC: American Psychiatric Press.

Strauss, J.S., Bowers, M., Downey, T.W., Fleck, S., Jackson, S., and Levine, I. (1980). *The psychotherapy of schizophrenia*. Northvale, NJ: Jason Aronson.

Suddath, R., Christison, G., Torrey, E., Casanova, M., and Weinberger, D. (1990). Anatomical abnormalities in the brains of monozygotic twins discordant for schizophrenia. *New England Journal of Medicine,* 322, 789-794.

Suranyi, L.K., and Jensen, G.D. (1993). *Trance and possession in Bali: A window on Western multiple personality, possession disorder, and suicide.* New York: Oxford University Press.

Swett, C., Surrey, J., and Cohen, C. (1990). Sexual and physical abuse histories and psychiatric symptoms among male psychiatric outpatients. *American Journal of Psychiatry,* 147, 632-636.

Szeszko, P.R., Strous, R.D., Goldman, R.S., Ashtari, M., Knuth, K.H., Lieberman, J.A., and Bilder, R.M. (2002). Neuropsychological correlates of hippocampal volumes in patients experiencing a first episode of schizophrenia. *American Journal of Psychiatry,* 159, 217-226.

Taiminen, T., Syvalahti, E., Saarijvari, S., Niemi, H., Lehto, H., Ahola, V., and Salokangas, R.K.R. (1997). Is positive placebo response in chronic schizophrenia investigator-dependent? *Journal of Nervous and Mental Disease,* 185, 644-645.

Tarrier, N., and Turpin, G. (1992). Psychosocial factors, arousal and schizophrenic relapse: The psychophysiological data. *British Journal of Psychiatry,* 161, 3-11.

Taylor, M.A., Berenbaum, S.A., Jampala, V.C., and Cloninger, C.R. (1993). Are schizophrenia and affective disorder related? Preliminary data from a family study. *American Journal of Psychiatry,* 150, 278-285.

Teuchert-Noodt, G. (2000). Neuronal degeneration and reorganization: A mutual principle in pathological and in healthy interactions of limbic and prefrontal circuits. *Journal of Neural Transmission,* 60 (Supplement), 315-333.

Thatcher, V.S., and McQueen, A. (1984). *The new Webster encyclopedic dictionary of the English language.* New York: Avenel Books.

Tice, P.P., Whittenburg, J.A., Baker, G.L., and Lemey, D.E. (2002). The real controversy about child sexual abuse research: Contradictory findings not addressed by Rind, Tromovitch, and Bauserman in their 1998 outcomes meta-analysis. *Journal of Child Sexual Abuse,* 9, 157-182.

Tienari, P. (1963). Psychiatric illnesses in identical twins. *Acta Psychiatrica Scandinavica,* 39 (Supplement 171), 10-195.

Tienari, P. (1991). Interaction between genetic vulnerability and family environment. *Acta Psychiatrica Scandinavica,* 84, 460-465.

Tienari, P., and Wynne, L. (1994). Adoption studies of schizophrenia. *Annals of Medicine,* 26, 233-237.

Torrey, E.F. (1992). Are we overestimating the genetic contribution to schizophrenia? *Schizophrenia Bulletin,* 18, 159-170.

Torrey, E.F., Bowler, A.E., Taylor, E.H., and Gottesman, I.I. (1994). *Schizophrenia and manic-depressive disorder.* New York: Perseus Books.

Tranter, R., O'Donovan, C., Chandarana, P., and Kennedy, S. (2002). Prevalence and outcome of partial remission in depression. *Journal of Psychiatry and Neuroscience,* 27, 241-247.

Tsuang, M.T., and Faraone, S.V. (2002). Diagnostic concepts and prevention of schizophrenia. *Canadian Journal of Psychiatry,* 47, 515-517.

Tsuang, M.T., Stone, W.S., and Faraone, S.V. (2000). Toward reformulating the diagnosis of schizophrenia. *American Journal of Psychiatry,* 157, 1041-1050.

Tsuang, M.T., Stone, W.S., and Faraone, S.V. (2002). Understanding predisposition to schizophrenia: Toward intervention and prevention. *Canadian Journal of Psychiatry,* 47, 518-526.

Turkheimer, E. (1998). Heritability and biological explanation. *Psychology Review,* 105, 782-791.

Turner, B.A. (1993). First-person account: The children of madness. *Schizophrenia Bulletin,* 19, 649-650.

Tutkun, H., Sar, V., Yargic, L.I., Ozpulat, T., Yanik, M., and Kizitlan, E. (1998). Frequency of dissociative disorders among psychiatric inpatients in a Turkish university clinic. *American Journal of Psychiatry,* 155, 800-805.

Van der Hart, O., and Friedman, B. (1989). A reader's guide to Pierre Janet on dissociation. *Dissociation,* 2, 3-16.

Van der Hart, O., Witztum, E., and Friedman, B. (1993). From hysterical psychosis to reactive dissociative psychosis. *Journal of Traumatic Stress,* 6, 43-64.

van der Kolk, B.A., McFarlane, A.C., and Weisath, L. (1996). *Traumatic stress: The effects of overwhelming experience on mind, body, and society.* New York: The Guilford Press.

van Erp, T.G.M., Saleh, P.A., Rosso, I.M., Huttunen, M., Lonnqvist, J., Pirkola, T., Salonen, O., Valanne, L., Poutanen, V.P., Standertskjold-Nordenstam, C.-G., et al. (2002). Contributions of genetic risk and fetal hypoxia to hippocampal volume in patients with schizophrenia or schizoaffective disorder, their unaffected siblings, and healthy unrelated controls. *American Journal of Psychiatry,* 159, 1514-1520.

Vanderlinden, J. (1993). *Dissociative experiences, trauma and hypnosis: Research findings and clinical applications in eating disorders.* Delft, Netherlands: Uitgeverij Eburon.

Vanderlinden, J., and Vandereycken, W. (1997). *Trauma, dissociation, and impulse dyscontrol in eating disorders.* Bristol, PA: Brunner/Mazel.

Villarreal, G., Petropoulos, H., Hamilton, D.A., Rowland, L.M., Horan, W.P., Griego, J.A., Moreshead, M., Hart, B.L., and Brooks, W.M. (2002). Proton magnetic resonance spectroscopy of the hippocampus and occipital white matter in PTSD: Preliminary results. *Canadian Journal of Psychiatry,* 47, 666-670.

Volavka, J., Czober, P., Sheitman, B., Lindenmayer, J.-P., Citrome, L., McEvoy, J.P., Cooper, T.B., Chakos, M., and Lieberman, J.A. (2002). Clozapine, olanzapine, risperidone, and haloperidol in the treatment of patients with chronic schizophrenia and schizoaffective disorder. *American Journal of Psychiatry,* 159, 255-262.

Volkmar, F. (1996). Childhood and adolescent psychosis: A review of the past 10 years. *Journal of the American Academy of Child and Adolescent Psychiatry,* 35, 843-851.

Waldfogel, S., and Mueser, K.T. (1988). Another case of chronic PTSD with auditory hallucinations. *American Journal of Psychiatry,* 145, 1314.

Waldinger, R.J., Swett, C., Frank, A., and Miller, K. (1994). Levels of dissociation and histories of reported abuse among women outpatients. *Journal of Nervous and Mental Disease*, 182, 625-630.

Walker, E., Cudbeck, R., Mednick, S., and Schlusinger, F. (1981). Effects of parental absence and institutionalization on the development of clinical symptoms in high-risk children. *Acta Psychiatrica Scandinavica*, 63, 95-109.

Walker, E., and Diforio, D. (1997). Schizophrenia: A neural diathesis-stress model. *Psychology Review*, 104, 667-685.

Walker, J.R., Norton, G.R., and Ross, C.A. (1991). *Panic disorder and agoraphobia: A comprehensive guide for the practitioner*. Pacific Grove, CA: Brooks/Cole.

Waller, N.G., Putnam, F.W., and Carlson, E.B. (1996). The types of dissociation and dissociative types: A taxometric analysis of dissociative experiences. *Psychological Methods*, 1, 300-321.

Waller, N.G., and Ross, C.A. (1997). The prevalence and biometric structure of pathological dissociation in the general population: Taxometric structure and behavior genetic findings. *Journal of Abnormal and Social Psychology*, 106, 499-510.

Walsh, B.T., Seidman, S.N., Sysko, R., and Gould, M. (2002). Placebo response in studies of major depression. *Journal of the American Medical Association*, 287, 1840-1847.

Whalen, J.E., and Nash, M.R. (1996). Hypnosis and dissociation: Theoretical, empirical, and clinical perspectives. In L.K. Michelson, and W.J. Ray (Eds.), *Handbook of dissociation: Theoretical, empirical, and clinical perspectives* (pp. 191-206). New York: Plenum.

Whitaker, R. (2001). *Mad in America: Bad science, bad medicine, and the enduring mistreatment of the mentally ill*. New York: Perseus.

Whitfield, C. (2002). The "false memory" defense: Using disinformation and junk science in and out of court. *Journal of Child Sexual Abuse*, 9, 53-78.

Whitfield, C.L., Silberg, J., and Fink, P.J. (2002). Introduction: Exposing misinformation concerning child sexual abuse and adult survivors. *Journal of Child Sexual Abuse*, 9, 1-8.

Whittenburg, J.A., Tice, P.P., Baker, G.L., and Lemmey, D.E. (2002). A critical appraisal of the 1998 meta-analytic review of child sexual abuse outcomes reported by Rind, Tromovitch, and Bauserman. *Journal of Child Sexual Abuse*, 9, 135-156.

Wilcox, J., Briones, D., and Suess, L. (1991). Auditory hallucinations, posttraumatic stress disorder, and ethnicity. *Comprehensive Psychiatry*, 32, 320-323.

Williams, L.M. (1994). Recall of childhood trauma: A prospective study of women's memories of child sexual abuse. *Journal of Consulting and Clinical Psychology*, 62, 1167-1176.

Williams-Keeler, L., Milliken, H., and Jones, B. (1994). Psychosis as precipitating trauma for PTSD: A treatment strategy. *American Journal of Orthopsychiatry*, 64, 493-498.

Wiseman, B. (1995). *Psychiatry: The ultimate betrayal*. Los Angeles: Freedom Publishing.

Wurr, J., and Partridge, I.M. (1996). The prevalence of a history of childhood sexual abuse in an acute adult inpatient population. *Child Abuse and Neglect,* 20, 867-872.

Wykes, T., Tarrier, N., and Lewis, S. (1998). *Outcome and innovation in psychological treatment of schizophrenia.* New York: John Wiley and Sons.

Yen, S., Shea, M.T., Battle, C.L., Johnson, D.M., Zlotnick, C., Dolan-Sewell, R., Skodol, A.E., Grilo, C.M., Gunderson, J.G., Sanislow, C.A., et al., (2002). Traumatic exposure and posttraumatic stress disorder in borderline, schizotypal, avoidant, and obsessive-compulsive personality disorders: Findings from a collaborative longitudinal personality disorders study. *Journal of Nervous and Mental Disease,* 190, 510-518.

Zahn, T.P., Moraga, R., and Ray, W.J. (1996). Psychophysiological assessment of dissociative disorders. In L.K. Michelson and W.J. Ray (Eds.), *Handbook of dissociation: Theoretical, empirical, and clinical perspectives* (pp. 269-290). New York: Plenum.

Zanarini, M.C., Frankenburg, F.R., Dubo, E.D., Sickel, A.E., Trikha, A., Levin, A., and Reynolds, V. (1998). Axis I comorbidity of borderline personality disorder. *American Journal of Psychiatry,* 155, 1733-1739.

Zanarini, M.C., Frankenburg, F.R., Hennen, J., and Silk, K.R. (2003). The longitudinal course of borderline psychopathology: 6-year prospective follow-up of the phenomenology of borderline personality disorder. *American Journal of Psychiatry,* 160, 274-283.

Zelikovsky, N., and Lynn, S.J. (2002). Childhood psychological and physical abuse: Psychopathology, dissociation, and Axis I diagnosis. *Journal of Trauma and Dissociation,* 3, 27-58.

Index

Page numbers followed by the letter "b" indicate boxed material; those followed by the letter "f" indicate figures; and those followed by the letter "t" indicate tables.

THE HAWORTH MALTREATMENT AND TRAUMA PRESS®
Robert A. Geffner, PhD
Senior Editor

SCHIZOPHRENIA: INNOVATIONS IN DIAGNOSIS AND TREATMENT by Colin A. Ross. (2004). "This book is a *must* for all clinicians and researchers dealing with serious mental disorders. Students in the various mental health disciplines are strongly recommended to read this book, thereby preventing themselves from copying traditional views that have been so detrimental to patients suffering from dissociative schizophrenia." *Onno van der Hart, PhD, Professor of Psychopathology of Chronic Traumatization, Utrecht University, Utrecht, the Netherlands*

MUNCHAUSEN BY PROXY: IDENTIFICATION, INTERVENTION, AND CASE MANAGEMENT by Louisa J. Lasher and Mary S. Sheridan. (2004). "This book is an excellent resource for professionals from all disciplines who may be confronted with this misunderstood disorder. Any question one would have regarding MSP—from the initial identification to assisting victim with treatment—is thoroughly addressed. This book is a must for every professional involved in MBP investigations." *Larry C. Brubaker, FBI Special Agent (retired)*

MOTHER-DAUGHTER INCEST: A GUIDE FOR HELPING PROFESSIONALS by Beverly A. Ogilvie. (2004). "Beverly A. Ogilvie has succeeded in writing what will become the definitive resource for therapists working with mother-daughter incest. Ogilvie presents a solid theoretical background, blending developmental, object-relations, self-in-relation, and attachment theories to explain the dynamics of this rare but devastating abuse. The book moves beyond theory and provides a working model to guide therapists working in this area." *Gina M. Pallotta, PhD, Associate Professor of Psychology and Clinical Graduate Director, California State University, Stanislaus*

REBUILDING ATTACHMENTS WITH TRAUMATIZED CHILDREN: HEALING FROM LOSSES, VIOLENCE, ABUSE, AND NEGLECT by Richard Kagan. (2004). "Dr. Richard Kagan, a recognized expert in working with traumatized children, has written a truly impressive book. Not only does the book contain a wealth of information for understanding the complex issues faced by traumatized youngsters, but it also offers specific interventions that can be used to help these children and their caregivers become more hopeful and resilient. . . . I am certain that this book will be read and reread by professionals engaged in improving the lives of at-risk youth." *Robert Brooks, PhD, Faculty, Harvard Medical School and author of* Raising Resilient Children *and* The Power of Resilience

PSYCHOLOGICAL TRAUMA AND THE DEVELOPING BRAIN: NEUROLOGICALLY BASED INTERVENTIONS FOR TROUBLED CHILDREN by Phyllis T. Stien and Joshua C. Kendall. (2003). "Stien and Kendall provide us with a great service. In this clearly written and important book, they synthesize a wealth of crucial information that links childhood trauma to brain abnormalities and subsequent mental illness. Equally important, they show us how the trauma also affects the child's social and intellectual development. I recommend this book to all clinicians and administrators." *Charles L. Whitfield, MD, Author of* The Truth About Depression *and* The Truth About Mental Illness

CHILD MALTREATMENT RISK ASSESSMENTS: AN EVALUATION GUIDE by Sue Righthand, Bruce Kerr, and Kerry Drach. (2003). "This book is essential reading for clinicians and forensic examiners who see cases involving issues related to child maltreatment. The authors have compiled an impressive critical survey of the relevant research on child maltreatment. Their material is well organized into sections on definitions, impact, risk assessment, and risk management. This book represents a giant step toward promoting evidence-based evaluations, treatment, and testimony." *Diane H. Schetky, MD, Professor of Psychiatry, University of Vermont College of Medicine*

SIMPLE AND COMPLEX POST-TRAUMATIC STRESS DISORDER: STRATEGIES FOR COMPREHENSIVE TREATMENT IN CLINICAL PRACTICE edited by Mary Beth Williams and John F. Sommer Jr. (2002). "A welcome addition to the literature on treating survivors of traumatic events, this volume possesses all the ingredients necessary for even the experienced clinician to master the management of patients with PTSD." *Terence M. Keane, PhD, Chief, Psychology Service, VA Boston Healthcare System; Professor and Vice Chair of Research in Psychiatry, Boston University School of Medicine*

FOR LOVE OF COUNTRY: CONFRONTING RAPE AND SEXUAL HARASSMENT IN THE U.S. MILITARY by T. S. Nelson. (2002). "Nelson brings an important message—that the absence of current media attention doesn't mean the problem has gone away; that only decisive action by military leadership at all levels can break the cycle of repeated traumatization; and that the failure to do so is, as Nelson puts it, a 'power failure'—a refusal to exert positive leadership at all levels to stop violent individuals from using the worst power imaginable." *Chris Lombardi, Correspondent, Women's E-News, New York City*

THE INSIDERS: A MAN'S RECOVERY FROM TRAUMATIC CHILDHOOD ABUSE by Robert Blackburn Knight. (2002). "An important book. . . . Fills a gap in the literature about healing from childhood sexual abuse by allowing us to hear, in undiluted terms, about one man's history and journey of recovery." *Amy Pine, MA, LMFT, psychotherapist and co-founder, Survivors Healing Center, Santa Cruz, California*

WE ARE NOT ALONE: A GUIDEBOOK FOR HELPING PROFESSIONALS AND PARENTS SUPPORTING ADOLESCENT VICTIMS OF SEXUAL ABUSE by Jade Christine Angelica. (2002). "Encourages victims and their families to participate in the system in an effort to heal from their victimization, seek justice, and hold offenders accountable for their crimes. An exceedingly vital training tool." *Janet Fine, MS, Director, Victim Witness Assistance Program and Children's Advocacy Center, Suffolk County District Attorney's Office, Boston*

WE ARE NOT ALONE: A TEENAGE GIRL'S PERSONAL ACCOUNT OF INCEST FROM DISCLOSURE THROUGH PROSECUTION AND TREATMENT by Jade Christine Angelica. (2002). "A valuable resource for teens who have been sexually abused and their parents. With compassion and eloquent prose, Angelica walks people through the criminal justice system—from disclosure to final outcome." *Kathleen Kendall-Tackett, PhD, Research Associate, Family Research Laboratory, University of New Hampshire, Durham*

WE ARE NOT ALONE: A TEENAGE BOY'S PERSONAL ACCOUNT OF CHILD SEXUAL ABUSE FROM DISCLOSURE THROUGH PROSECUTION AND TREATMENT by Jade Christine Angelica. (2002). "Inspires us to work harder to meet kids' needs, answer their questions, calm their fears, and protect them from their abusers and the system, which is often not designed to respond to them in a language they understand." *Kevin L. Ryle, JD, Assistant District Attorney, Middlesex, Massachusetts*

GROWING FREE: A MANUAL FOR SURVIVORS OF DOMESTIC VIOLENCE by Wendy Susan Deaton and Michael Hertica. (2001). "This is a necessary book for anyone who is scared and starting to think about what it would take to 'grow free.' . . . Very helpful for friends and relatives of a person in a domestic violence situation. I recommend it highly." *Colleen Friend, LCSW, Field Work Consultant, UCLA Department of Social Welfare, School of Public Policy & Social Research*

A THERAPIST'S GUIDE TO GROWING FREE: A MANUAL FOR SURVIVORS OF DOMESTIC VIOLENCE by Wendy Susan Deaton and Michael Hertica. (2001). "An excellent synopsis of the theories and research behind the manual." *Beatrice Crofts Yorker, RN, JD, Professor of Nursing, Georgia State University, Decatur*

PATTERNS OF CHILD ABUSE: HOW DYSFUNCTIONAL TRANSACTIONS ARE REPLICATED IN INDIVIDUALS, FAMILIES, AND THE CHILD WELFARE SYSTEM by Michael Karson. (2001). "No one interested in what may well be the major public health epidemic of our time in terms of its long-term consequences for our society can afford to pass up the opportunity to read this enlightening work." *Howard Wolowitz, PhD, Professor Emeritus, Psychology Department, University of Michigan, Ann Arbor*

IDENTIFYING CHILD MOLESTERS: PREVENTING CHILD SEXUAL ABUSE BY RECOGNIZING THE PATTERNS OF THE OFFENDERS by Carla van Dam. (2000). "The definitive work on the subject. . . . Provides parents and others with the tools to recognize when and how to intervene." *Roger W. Wolfe, MA, Co-Director, N. W. Treatment Associates, Seattle, Washington*

POLITICAL VIOLENCE AND THE PALESTINIAN FAMILY: IMPLICATIONS FOR MENTAL HEALTH AND WELL-BEING by Vivian Khamis. (2000). "A valuable book . . . a pioneering work that fills a glaring gap in the study of Palestinian society." *Elia Zureik, Professor of Sociology, Queens University, Kingston, Ontario, Canada*

STOPPING THE VIOLENCE: A GROUP MODEL TO CHANGE MEN'S ABUSIVE ATTITUDES AND BEHAVIORS by David J. Decker. (1999). "A concise and thorough manual to assist clinicians in learning the causes and dynamics of domestic violence." *Joanne Kittel, MSW, LICSW, Yachats, Oregon*

STOPPING THE VIOLENCE: A GROUP MODEL TO CHANGE MEN'S ABUSIVE ATTITUDES AND BEHAVIORS, THE CLIENT WORKBOOK by David J. Decker. (1999).

BREAKING THE SILENCE: GROUP THERAPY FOR CHILDHOOD SEXUAL ABUSE, A PRACTITIONER'S MANUAL by Judith A. Margolin. (1999). "This book is an extremely valuable and well-written resource for all therapists working with adult survivors of child sexual abuse." *Esther Deblinger, PhD, Associate Professor of Clinical Psychiatry, University of Medicine and Dentistry of New Jersey School of Osteopathic Medicine*

"I NEVER TOLD ANYONE THIS BEFORE": MANAGING THE INITIAL DISCLOSURE OF SEXUAL ABUSE RE-COLLECTIONS by Janice A. Gasker. (1999). "Discusses the elements needed to create a safe, therapeutic environment and offers the practitioner a number of useful strategies for responding appropriately to client disclosure." *Roberta G. Sands, PhD, Associate Professor, University of Pennsylvania School of Social Work*

FROM SURVIVING TO THRIVING: A THERAPIST'S GUIDE TO STAGE II RECOVERY FOR SURVIVORS OF CHILDHOOD ABUSE by Mary Bratton. (1999). "A must read for all, including survivors. Bratton takes a lifelong debilitating disorder and unravels its intricacies in concise, succinct, and understandable language." *Phillip A. Whitner, PhD, Sr. Staff Counselor, University Counseling Center, The University of Toledo, Ohio*

SIBLING ABUSE TRAUMA: ASSESSMENT AND INTERVENTION STRATEGIES FOR CHILDREN, FAMILIES, AND ADULTS by John V. Caffaro and Allison Conn-Caffaro. (1998). "One area that has almost consistently been ignored in the research and writing on child maltreatment is the area of sibling abuse. This book is a welcome and required addition to the developing literature on abuse." *Judith L. Alpert, PhD, Professor of Applied Psychology, New York University*

BEARING WITNESS: VIOLENCE AND COLLECTIVE RESPONSIBILITY by Sandra L. Bloom and Michael Reichert. (1998). "A totally convincing argument. . . . Demands careful study by all elected representatives, the clergy, the mental health and medical professions, representatives of the media, and all those unwittingly involved in this repressive perpetuation and catastrophic global problem." *Harold I. Eist, MD, Past President, American Psychiatric Association*

TREATING CHILDREN WITH SEXUALLY ABUSIVE BEHAVIOR PROBLEMS: GUIDELINES FOR CHILD AND PARENT INTERVENTION by Jan Ellen Burton, Lucinda A. Rasmussen, Julie Bradshaw, Barbara J. Christopherson, and Steven C. Huke. (1998). "An extremely readable book that is well-documented and a mine of valuable 'hands on' information. . . . This is a book that all those who work with sexually abusive children or want to work with them must read." *Sharon K. Araji, PhD, Professor of Sociology, University of Alaska, Anchorage*

THE LEARNING ABOUT MYSELF (LAMS) PROGRAM FOR AT-RISK PARENTS: LEARNING FROM THE PAST—CHANGING THE FUTURE by Verna Rickard. (1998). "This program should be a part of the resource materials of every mental health professional trusted with the responsibility of working with 'at-risk' parents." *Terry King, PhD, Clinical Psychologist, Federal Bureau of Prisons, Catlettsburg, Kentucky*

THE LEARNING ABOUT MYSELF (LAMS) PROGRAM FOR AT-RISK PARENTS: HANDBOOK FOR GROUP PARTICIPANTS by Verna Rickard. (1998). "Not only is the LAMS program designed to be educational and build skills for future use, it is also fun!" *Martha Morrison Dore, PhD, Associate Professor of Social Work, Columbia University, New York*

BRIDGING WORLDS: UNDERSTANDING AND FACILITATING ADOLESCENT RECOVERY FROM THE TRAUMA OF ABUSE by Joycee Kennedy and Carol McCarthy. (1998). "An extraordinary survey of the history of child neglect and abuse in America. . . . A wonderful teaching tool at the university level, but should be required reading in high schools as well." *Florabel Kinsler, PhD, BCD, LCSW, Licensed Clinical Social Worker, Los Angeles, California*

CEDAR HOUSE: A MODEL CHILD ABUSE TREATMENT PROGRAM by Bobbi Kendig with Clara Lowry. (1998). "Kendig and Lowry truly . . . realize the saying that we are our brothers' keepers. Their spirit permeates this volume, and that spirit of caring is what always makes the difference for people in painful situations." *Hershel K. Swinger, PhD, Clinical Director, Children's Institute International, Los Angeles, California*

SEXUAL, PHYSICAL, AND EMOTIONAL ABUSE IN OUT-OF-HOME CARE: PRE-VENTION SKILLS FOR AT-RISK CHILDREN by Toni Cavanagh Johnson and Associates. (1997). "Professionals who make dispositional decisions or who are related to out-of-home care for children could benefit from reading and following the curriculum of this book with children in placements." *Issues in Child Abuse Accusations*

Order a copy of this book with this form or online at:
http://www.haworthpress.com/store/product.asp?sku=5107

SCHIZOPHRENIA
Innovations in Diagnosis and Treatment

_____in hardbound at $49.95 (ISBN: 0-7890-2269-9)

_____in softbound at $34.95 (ISBN: 0-7890-2270-2)

Or order online and use special offer code HEC25 in the shopping cart.

COST OF BOOKS_____

POSTAGE & HANDLING_____
(US: $4.00 for first book & $1.50
for each additional book)
(Outside US: $5.00 for first book
& $2.00 for each additional book)

SUBTOTAL_____

IN CANADA: ADD 7% GST_____

STATE TAX_____
(NY, OH, MN, CA, IL, IN, & SD residents,
add appropriate local sales tax)

FINAL TOTAL_____
(If paying in Canadian funds,
convert using the current
exchange rate, UNESCO
coupons welcome)

☐ **BILL ME LATER:** (Bill-me option is good on
US/Canada/Mexico orders only; not good to
jobbers, wholesalers, or subscription agencies.)
☐ Check here if billing address is different from
shipping address and attach purchase order and
billing address information.

Signature_____

☐ **PAYMENT ENCLOSED: $_____**

☐ **PLEASE CHARGE TO MY CREDIT CARD.**

☐ Visa ☐ MasterCard ☐ AmEx ☐ Discover
☐ Diner's Club ☐ Eurocard ☐ JCB

Account # _____

Exp. Date_____

Signature_____

Prices in US dollars and subject to change without notice.

NAME_____

INSTITUTION_____

ADDRESS_____

CITY_____

STATE/ZIP_____

COUNTRY_____ COUNTY (NY residents only)_____

TEL_____ FAX_____

E-MAIL_____

May we use your e-mail address for confirmations and other types of information? ☐ Yes ☐ No
We appreciate receiving your e-mail address and fax number. Haworth would like to e-mail or fax special
discount offers to you, as a preferred customer. **We will never share, rent, or exchange your e-mail address
or fax number.** We regard such actions as an invasion of your privacy.

Order From Your Local Bookstore or Directly From
The Haworth Press, Inc.
10 Alice Street, Binghamton, New York 13904-1580 • USA
TELEPHONE: 1-800-HAWORTH (1-800-429-6784) / Outside US/Canada: (607) 722-5857
FAX: 1-800-895-0582 / Outside US/Canada: (607) 771-0012
E-mailto: orders@haworthpress.com

For orders outside US and Canada, you may wish to order through your local
sales representative, distributor, or bookseller.
For information, see http://haworthpress.com/distributors

(Discounts are available for individual orders in US and Canada only, not booksellers/distributors.)

PLEASE PHOTOCOPY THIS FORM FOR YOUR PERSONAL USE.
http://www.HaworthPress.com   BOF04

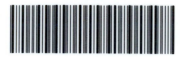
DATE DUE

JUL 1 1 2007		
APR 2 2 2009		
MAR 3 1 2009		
MAR 3 1 2010		
MAR 3 1 2010		
MAR 3 0 2011		
APR 2 0 2011		
APR 2 1 2011		
MAY 1 6 2014		
MAY 1 3 2014		
GAYLORD		PRINTED IN U.S.A.